MEDICAL NOTES FOR SOCIAL WORKERS

FRADA ESKIN, M.B., Ch.B.,
D.Obst., R.C.O.G.

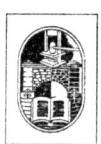

BRISTOL: JOHN WRIGHT & SONS LTD.
1971

© Frada Eskin 1971

All Rights Reserved. No part of this publication may be reproduced, stored in a retrieval system, or transmitted, in any form or by any means, electronic, mechanical, photocopying, recording or otherwise, without the prior permission of John Wright & Sons Ltd.

Distribution by Sole Agents:
United States of America: The Williams & Wilkins Company,
Baltimore
Canada: The Macmillan Company of Canada Ltd., Toronto

ISBN 0 7236 0306 5

PRINTED IN GREAT BRITAIN
BY JOHN WRIGHT & SONS LTD.
AT THE STONEBRIDGE PRESS, BRISTOL

To my husband and parents

PREFACE

Chronic illness leading to disability may also be responsible for emotional disturbance, requiring the expertise of a social caseworker. However, it must be remembered that the observed emotional disorder may be an integral part of the medical disorder and will not be alleviated by casework technique. A detailed knowledge of medicine is not necessary for social workers dealing with the problems of the disabled, but it is important that they should be aware of the basic facts concerning chronic diseases so that their clients may best be served.

Emotional problems may arise owing to several factors. The alteration in circumstances often necessitated by the onset of disability may cause conflict in a variety of ways, depending upon the original circumstances of the person afflicted by illness. The emotional upheaval engendered by conflict may aggravate the medical condition which in turn further increases conflict. A man who has been the bread-winner and sole supporter of his family may find it difficult to adjust to changes which may include loss of roles as wage-earner, father, and husband, and his wife may be unable to adjust to the new situation, particularly if she is forced to assume the responsibility for the economic support of her family. In this type of situation other factors have to be taken into consideration before the problems may be tackled adequately. The disease initiating conflict may do so directly by affecting brain tissue and causing damage to the part of the brain responsible for the control of emotional responses. In some chronic illnesses, toxic substances are formed in the diseased tissues which may act directly on the brain and cause personality changes as well as physical symptoms. If the social caseworker has some knowledge of the illness that is being dealt with, he or she is more likely to arrive at an accurate assessment of the presenting situation.

There are several different types of chronic disease that may cause permanent disability. There are those conditions which cause destruction of tissue at one point in time with no further damage, and in fact there may be some limited improvement with the passage of time, e.g., poliomyelitis, stroke, loss of limbs due to accident, and cerebral palsy. There are also those diseases which are termed progressive, and which in general continue to attack an increasing proportion of body tissue until death ensues. Occasionally there is an arrest of progress, but in most cases this does not occur, e.g., multiple sclerosis, muscular dystrophy, and Friedreich's ataxia. There are some diseases which progress until a large portion of body tissue is destroyed and then appear to burn themselves out, e.g., rheumatoid arthritis. There are other chronic diseases which have acute periods followed by quiescent periods during which the person may be relatively well for some years. However, each time an acute episode of the condition occurs this leads to further tissue damage until finally there is permanent ill health, e.g., asthma and chronic bronchitis, coronary heart disease, and epilepsy. Other chronic diseases may be controlled to an extent which enables the person to lead a healthy life. However, the control is often finely balanced and a careful check has to be maintained, e.g., diabetes, thyrotoxicosis, and hypertension.

In this book I have tried to describe the common chronic conditions which may be encountered. Although I have described basic symptoms, prognosis, and treatment, I have also attempted to indicate the way in which a particular disease may affect the person as a whole in his daily life. I have, in addition, included subjects concerned with health and disease which a social worker may come across in his or her daily contact with the chronically sick.

I would like to thank Mrs. P. Krausz and Mr. E. Wilkinson, who spent a great deal of time reading my manuscript and correcting my many mistakes.

1971　　　　　　　　　　　　　　　　　　　F. Eskin

CONTENTS

	PAGE		PAGE
Addison's Disease	9	Friedreich's Ataxia	51
Alcoholism	9	Gall-stones	52
Amputation	11	Gastric Ulcer	53
Anaemia	13	Glaucoma	54
Anxiety	14	Gonorrhoea	55
Asthma	16	Haemophilia	57
Barbiturates	17	Hay Fever	58
B.C.G.	19	The Heart	59
Bed-sores	20	Hodgkin's Disease	60
Bronchiectasis	22	Hormones	61
Bronchitis	24	Huntington's Chorea	61
Cancer	25	Hydrocephalus	62
Cardiac Arrest	27	Hypertension	64
Cataract	28	Hypothermia	65
Catheter	29	Ichthyosis	66
Cerebral Palsy	30	Ileal Loop	67
Cerebral Thrombosis	31	Incontinence of Urine	68
Cholesterol	33	Influenza	70
Christmas Disease	33	Insulin	71
Coronary Heart Disease	34	Iron	73
Crohn's Disease	36	Jaundice	74
Cushing's Syndrome	37	The Kidney	75
Deafness	38	Leprosy	76
Diabetes Mellitus	40	Leukaemia	77
Down's Syndrome	42	Lungs	78
Drug Addiction	43	Multiple Sclerosis	79
Eczema	45	Muscular Dystrophy	81
Emphysema	46	Myasthenia Gravis	82
Enuresis	47	Myxoedema	83
Epilepsy	48	Nephritis	84
Flatulence	50	Obesity	85

	PAGE		PAGE
OEDEMA	87	SMOKING	103
OSTEO-ARTHRITIS	88	SODIUM	104
PARAPLEGIA	89	SPINA BIFIDA	105
THE PITUITARY GLAND	91	SYPHILIS	106
POLIOMYELITIS	92	THRUSH	108
POTASSIUM	94	THYROTOXICOSIS	109
PSORIASIS	95	TUBERCULOSIS	110
PULMONARY EMBOLUS	96	ULCERATIVE COLITIS	112
QUINSY	97	URTICARIA	114
RENAL DIALYSIS	97	VARICOSE VEINS	114
RHEUMATIC FEVER	99	VITAMINS	116
RHEUMATOID ARTHRITIS	100	WHOOPING-COUGH	117
		YAWS	118
SMALL-POX	101	YELLOW FEVER	119

MEDICAL NOTES FOR SOCIAL WORKERS

ADDISON'S DISEASE

Addison's disease is due to failure of function of the adrenal glands. The adrenal glands are situated, one on each side of the body, just above the kidneys and consist of two parts, cortex and medulla. The symptoms of Addison's disease are due to destruction of the adrenal cortex. In some cases the damage is due to tuberculosis infection. However, in the majority of cases there is no obvious cause for tissue destruction. The adrenal cortex produces hormones which regulate carbohydrate metabolism, assist the utilization of sodium and potassium by the body, and control sexual function and growth. All the symptoms of Addison's disease are due to failure of production of these hormones and include extreme tiredness, pigmentation of the skin, low blood-pressure, vomiting and diarrhoea, and loss of weight. Other diseases are often associated with Addison's disease. These include diabetes mellitus and pernicious anaemia. Treatment is by replacement therapy and any extra strain on the body, such as operations or infections, must be covered by extra dosage of adrenal cortical hormones. With modern treatment life expectancy has improved and with care anyone affected by this condition can now live a normal life-span.

ALCOHOLISM

Alcoholism may be defined as an addiction to alcohol. Severe physical symptoms occur when alcohol is no longer available to the individual dependent upon this drug.

Social, physical, and psychological reasons equally may be incriminated for the development of the addictive state. Many people drink socially but never become dependent on alcohol. Only certain personalities are 'at risk' in this context. Some people need alcohol to allay their anxieties, to help them to be sociable, or to relax their inhibitions from the sexual point of view. People who have inadequate personalities and who find it difficult to cope with daily life are most likely to find alcohol a comfort, and then a necessity. Sometimes persons suffering with a painful physical condition drink alcohol to relieve pain and may develop a dependence if the physical condition is chronic. It is also considered that the tendency to alcoholism may be inherited in some people and that these individuals are more likely to succumb when alcohol is available.

Addiction to alcohol leads to degeneration of mind and body and may cause early death. Alcoholics may be identified by a conglomeration of symptoms, some or all of which may be present. They may show slurred speech and shaky limbs, loss of memory, and degeneration in personal habits. Alcoholism gives rise to male impotence and this, in turn, leads to jealousy, aggression, and marital disharmony. As the alcoholic state continues, there may be attacks of delirium when the person becomes confused, disorientated, and has hallucinations. The end-results of prolonged addiction to alcoholism are extremely unpleasant. The chronic alcoholic drinks alone and in secret. He cannot do without an early morning drink. Because he is preoccupied with alcohol he forgets to eat; he loses weight and signs of liver damage due to alcoholic poisoning begin to appear. Lack of food intake also leads to lack of intake of essential substances, such as vitamins and minerals. Because of the lack of vitamins and minerals specific deficiency diseases may occur. Liver damage leading to cirrhosis of the liver (degeneration of liver tissue) gives rise to tremor of the limbs and damage to nerves. The damaged nerves produce loss of use and sensation in the limbs and other parts of the body. There are also severe mental changes, including loss of memory—particularly for recent events (Korsakow's syndrome).

Treating this disease is very difficult. The important factor is to gain the confidence of the person as treatment is most successful with a willing patient. Withdrawal of alcohol must coincide with drug treatment to alleviate the withdrawal symptoms. The person should be heavily sedated during the first 24 hours of treatment. Rehabilitation is most difficult as it is easy to succumb to old habits and return to alcohol. One drink is sufficient to destroy several months of intensive medical help. If possible a new life should be designed, with new surroundings, a new job, and different hobbies. It is essential to have the support of close relatives, as without this the treatment will fail. It is also important to try to discover the underlying reasons for the initial development of addiction and to see if these may be overcome. The success rate is low.

There is an organization called Alcoholics Anonymous, which consists of people who have been cured, who meet to give each other help and support following treatment. This is a good supportive organization, but once again does not guarantee a 100 per cent cure rate. In any family situation when either parent is suffering from alcoholism there are many problems associated with the children of that family, and the whole family situation will be affected when the individual is receiving intensive long-term help. Family counselling carried out early in the treatment may prevent the development of emotional and psychological difficulties in the children of the affected family.

AMPUTATION

The removal of limbs or organs due to accident, injury, or disease is referred to as amputation. However, for the purpose of this discussion, amputation will refer to the removal of limbs. When the blood-supply to a limb is reduced or completely cut off, the tissue no longer receives any nutrition and therefore dies. Death of tissue leads to gangrene and, as bacterial infection may complicate the whole process, it becomes necessary to amputate the dead tissue to prevent further damage. The dying and diseased tissue also causes a great deal of pain.

An accident or injury leading to amputation is usually so severe that the blood-supply to the limb is irrevocably damaged. Sometimes the blood-supply may be intact, but the tissue may be so severely damaged and crushed that it cannot be reconstructed and must be removed. Severe damage such as this may occur in a vehicle accident or in industrial injury.

There are several diseases responsible for affecting the blood-supply to limbs. The most common is atherosclerosis (hardening of the arteries). In this condition the main arteries become thickened and narrowed, and the blood-supply is reduced to various parts of the body, particularly to the legs. Walking may become painful (intermittent claudication) and sometimes, in the most severe cases, there is pain in the legs when the patient is resting. Tissue destruction is usually a slow process and it may be months or years before amputation is necessary. However, it sometimes happens that arteries already narrowed by disease may suddenly become completely blocked by a blood-clot, which causes sudden cessation of blood-supply and immediate tissue death. This condition usually requires amputation unless the clot can be removed immediately. Diabetes is often associated with atherosclerosis and the diabetic condition is thought to encourage the development of blood-vessel damage. There are many people with diabetes who have also had limbs amputated. Another disease of the blood-vessels, which is more acute and due to an inflammatory process, is known as Burgher's disease. This disease affects the blood-vessels and closes them, thus causing lack of blood-supply to the tissues and consequent tissue death. The disease is progressive and amputation of several limbs or parts of limbs may occur before the disease process burns itself out.

It is often very difficult to adjust to the loss of limbs, particularly in the older age-group. Losing part of the body, while not incompatible with life, makes some people feel less than whole human beings in a much wider sense than merely physical loss. The body-image is damaged. Adaptation always takes time and in some cases never occurs. The use of artificial limbs is more difficult in later life and lack of ability to use prostheses may lead to permanent wheel-chair existence. This increases the load placed on relatives and may cause marital conflict or increase that already present.

Amputation due to injury is a static condition and often occurs in young people as a result of motor-cycle and car accidents. Young people may feel more bitter at the time of the accident, but with youth on their side often make a good adjustment to the disability. In the older person, amputation is often due to a progressive disease process, where the outlook is poor and further amputation envisaged, complicating the problems of adaptation. However, adjustment to disability depends mainly on the personality of the person and the support received from friends and relatives. Intensive preparation prior to amputation is equally as important as the actual medical procedure if the end-result is to be an adequate and happy adjustment to an inevitable occurrence.

ANAEMIA

One of the main functions of the blood is to carry oxygen to the tissues. Oxygen is an essential requirement for the maintenance of life. If the normal oxygen-carrying power of the blood is reduced from whatever cause, the term given to the resulting condition is 'anaemia'. The blood contains red blood-cells which are responsible for carrying oxygen from the lungs to the tissues. Red blood-cells contain a complicated chemical substance called haemoglobin. Oxygen attaches itself to haemoglobin and is carried to the tissues. When oxygen reaches its destination, it becomes dissociated from haemoglobin, leaves the blood-stream, and can be utilized by the body. If the haemoglobin content of the blood is reduced, then the oxygen-carrying power is also reduced. The normal content of haemoglobin in the body is between 14 and 16 g. for every 100 ml. of blood. An arbitrary scale has been developed to measure haemoglobin levels in the body: 100 per cent represents 14·8 g. per 100 ml. When the percentage levels of haemoglobin fall below the accepted norm, the norm depending on sex, age, and physical condition of the individual, the person is said to be anaemic.

Reduced oxygen-carrying power of the blood may be due to several causes. Blood may be lost from the body (haemorrhage), blood-cells may be improperly formed and therefore break up easily, or there is abnormal destruction of red blood-cells in the blood-vessels (haemolysis). Anaemia due to acute haemorrhage may occur from injury or disease. Sometimes there is a chronic source of bleeding which, although only slight, gives rise over several years to chronic anaemia, e.g., piles (or haemorrhoids) and gastric ulcers. Haemophilia is an inherited disease with spontaneous haemorrhages occurring due to abnormalities of the clotting mechanism of the blood, and this disease can give rise to repeated episodes of acute severe anaemia. Anaemia may also be caused by haemolysis or abnormal destruction of the cells, which may be due to various poisons which enter the body. Transfusion of incompatible blood, snake-bites, and some bacterial poisons may cause haemolysis. Congenital conditions also exist with the formation of abnormal blood-cells by the blood-forming organs. These blood-cells are not as stable or as strong as normal blood-cells, e.g., sickle-cell anaemia. Lack of essential substances which are required for the formation of blood may cause anaemia. These include iron and vitamin B_{12}. Deficiency of one or more of these substances encourages abnormal blood-cell formation. Blood-cells are formed in the bone-marrow which must also be functioning normally for the production of normal cells. Any disease of bone-marrow will give rise to anaemia, e.g., leukaemia. Many acute and chronic illnesses affect the blood-forming organs probably due to the production of poisons by the disease processes, e.g., rheumatoid arthritis, tuberculosis, and severe skin conditions.

The symptoms associated with anaemia are similar whatever the cause. Breathlessness, tiredness, oedema (swelling due to retention of excess fluid), palpitation, depression, pallor, and cerebral confusion are all indicative of anaemia. Heart symptoms such as palpitation are due to the fact that the lack of oxygen stimulates an increased heart-rate in order to bring a larger supply of blood more quickly to tissues starved of oxygen. Lack of iron has particular symptoms, including a smooth and moist tongue, changes in the nails, and dyspepsia. Many of the symptoms of anaemia may be vague and ill-defined. Women are more prone to anaemic conditions due to menstruation and child-bearing, and are also more likely to be accused of neurotic behaviour. It is important to exclude anaemia and other organic diseases before instituting psychiatric treatment for neurotic symptoms. Removal of the cause of anaemia usually removes the symptoms and treats the condition.

ANXIETY

In considering anxiety as an abnormal and harmful condition one is not talking about the type of anxiety which besets everyone at some period of their lives, when involved in a new and difficult situation. In times of stress, anxiety symptoms occur in most normal people and in fact one always suspects an individual who shows no signs of disturbance when in the face of some alarming or difficult occurrence. Many situations provoke anxiety, depending to some extent on the basic personality of the individual. Pre-examination and pre-wedding nerves, change of job, or meeting new people are all prone to arouse normal anxiety feelings. However, there are certain situations which may, over a prolonged period, produce exaggerated anxiety responses which do not cease when the stress causing the symptoms is removed. Difficulties with a marriage partner or continual upset at work may provoke such an abnormal response and it is the occurrence of symptoms in these situations which are known as 'anxiety' in medical terminology.

Anxiety symptoms may include unreasonable fear, trembling, palpitations, sweating, and breathlessness. In severe cases there is anorexia (loss of appetite) and consequent loss of weight. Many of the symptoms associated with anxiety also occur in organic disease and the possibility of such disease must be excluded before a diagnosis of anxiety neurosis is made. Anxiety is a condition which may exist as long as the individual lives and which is exacerbated when he or she is exposed to those situations which trigger off the mechanism. For example, some people find that sitting in an enclosed place, such as a theatre or a cinema, gives them acute anxiety symptoms; as soon as they are able to leave, they feel well again. Such people have to sit at the end of a row so that they can make their escape should their symptoms arise.

Most people, once they realize the significance of their alarming symptoms, learn to cope with this disability and to overcome the feelings of anxiety when they occur. However, although this is a disturbance of the psyche, the symptoms are very real and the person can feel extremely ill. Mind and body are interdependent and it is thought that prolonged anxiety symptoms, while not indicative of organic disease, may eventually damage organs. However, this is merely surmise as yet and has not been proved. Anxiety symptoms superimposed on already damaged and diseased organs may provoke further damage.

It is important to give professional help as early as possible in any anxiety state, since early treatment may prevent development of the chronic anxiety state. Both the medical profession and social workers can aid a person to learn to live with his anxiety. The doctor can help by reassurance that all is well with the body and by prescribing sedatives and tranquillizers. The social worker, with knowledge of this condition, can help the individual to understand and to come to terms with himself as a human being.

ASTHMA

This is a condition affecting the respiratory system. The main effect is on the passages leading to the lungs from the external air, which are known as bronchi and bronchioles. These passages consist mainly of muscle tissue. During an asthmatic attack the nerves supplying this muscle cause excessive constriction of the bronchi and bronchioles. This prevents expiration of air from the lungs, which become distended and cause acute respiratory distress in the afflicted individual.

The disease is common in children and may persist into adolescence and adulthood. It is often associated with eczema (*see* ECZEMA). There is an inherited tendency to develop one or both of these conditions and the disease tends to run in families and to be associated with other allergic respiratory conditions such as hay fever.

The characteristic symptoms include wheezing and breathlessness, cough, and acute general distress. The cough, which is at first dry, becomes wet with the production of large quantities of sputum. Very occasionally one attack follows so quickly upon another that it becomes a single prolonged episode, dangerous to life and known as status asthmaticus. Asthmatic attacks are worse in the pre-pubertal boy or girl and often improve after the child passes puberty.

It used to be considered that asthma was triggered by emotional situations, but more recent research indicates that the cause of the attacks is more likely to be an allergic response to dust and pollen particles. These may include house dust, animal hairs, and other small particles carried in the atmosphere.

It has been said that the asthmatic child is highly emotional and hypersensitive. It is certainly true that a child suffering from frequent asthmatic attacks loses appetite and fails to thrive, giving the appearance of a frail and puny individual. Frequent absences from school, overprotection by parents, and difficulties with school friends may give rise in themselves to emotional conflicts (particularly where eczema coexists), and these are more likely the result and not the cause of the asthmatic bouts. However, any emotional conflict that is present will aggravate the effect of the allergic condition causing asthma. In many cases children with asthma have been shown to have a higher intelligence than average, although their work is limited due to frequent absences from school.

In an acute attack the obvious treatment is to relax the muscle tissue and this is achieved by various muscle-relaxant drugs. Cortisone and related compounds have an immediate relieving effect but should be used carefully. Increased use of aerosol cortisone sprays has been incriminated in the increase in numbers of sudden deaths during asthmatic attacks. Antibiotics are important in the treatment of attacks, since the asthmatic state leads to a weakening of resistance to bacterial attacks in lung tissue and consequent secondary infection.

It is difficult to give advice when counselling parents anxious to save any future progeny the distress of asthma and all the attendant complications. However, there is an inherited tendency to develop asthma and this must be taken into consideration when advising parents and looking at the family situation as a whole.

Older people with chronic chest conditions may develop asthmatic attacks. These are secondary to the chronic respiratory disease already present and such attacks are stimulated by the poisons produced in the system by diseases such as chronic bronchitis and emphysema. These attacks are best dealt with by treating the primary disease. Muscle relaxants may give immediate relief.

BARBITURATES

Most people are familiar with the group of drugs known as barbiturates, mainly in association with the problem of insomnia. Although many of this group have been in use since the beginning of the twentieth century, they are still popular with the medical profession and are prescribed in large amounts to middle-aged and elderly people of both sexes who complain of persistent sleeplessness.

These drugs all have a similar effect and vary mainly in the length of their action and the strength of action dose to dose. They are usually taken in tablet form, but when rapid action is required some can be given by injection directly into the blood-stream. Because the drugs of this group induce sleep they are known as hypnotics. However, some are also very effective in damping down or preventing epileptic fits. Sodium phenobarbitone is used extensively in the treatment of epilepsy. They are also used to treat convulsions due to other causes such as brain injury or brain disease.

Relief of pain is another property of the barbiturate group of drugs. However, larger doses are required for this effect since they are only mildly analgesic and are not used to relieve severe persistent pain. Some of this group are used in combination with other drugs to provide general anaesthesia and have become popular for this technique. For example, barbiturates are used for general anaesthesia in dental extractions.

Barbiturates act directly on the respiratory centre in the brain. Normally the respiratory centre reacts to the carbon dioxide content of the blood. The more carbon dioxide present the faster and deeper the respiratory rate and vice versa. Under the influence of barbiturates the respiratory centre becomes insensitive to carbon dioxide concentration in the blood. But it is still sensitive to oxygen concentrations and a low oxygen concentration in the blood stimulates respiration. In the treatment of barbiturate poisoning oxygen should not be given since it will cause further depression of the respiratory centre in the brain and breathing will cease.

Some drugs reinforce the effect of barbiturates. Caution is always required with alcohol intake if barbiturates are also being taken. A moderate dose, calculated for sedative effect only, can cause drowsiness if taken in conjunction with alcohol. This is particularly dangerous if driving is involved and anyone taking barbiturates should be warned of this danger. Barbiturates cause death by depressing the higher nerve centres including the vital functions of respiration and circulation.

Barbiturate overdose is a relatively pleasant method of suicide. There are no conscious painful effects, sleep occurs fairly rapidly and becomes gradually deeper until a state of coma exists. Finally, all vital functions cease and death occurs. It is easy to acquire barbiturates since at the present time they are generously prescribed for sleeping and stress problems. This is not the place in which to enter into a long dissertation of the ethics of revival of suicide victims. However, if an individual is suffering from a severely disabling and incurable disease and chooses to solve the problem in this way, should others refuse him the right to do so? Anyone who has suffered severe prolonged pain will appreciate the feelings of an individual who decides that suicide is the only course of action that will give permanent relief.

Members of the barbiturate group are still the most effective drugs for the problem of insomnia for many people. However, they should be used with caution since prolonged use may lead to addiction.

B.C.G.

These initials refer to a vaccine which is effective in the protection of human beings against infection by the tuberculosis bacteria. The vaccine is known as Bacille Calmette-Guérin and is of French origin. It is made from live tuberculosis bacteria, which have been processed so that they no longer cause harmful disease but can still act to give protection against infection by the more virulent natural strains of tuberculosis organisms.

Many people are attacked by the tuberculosis bacteria in their youth. In most cases the body defences are sufficient to overcome any bacterial invasion, others are never infected. Those who are, produce substances known as antibodies in response to the presence of the bacteria in the tissues. These antibodies remain in the bloodstream and if there is a further invasion by tuberculosis bacteria at some later stage, these bacteria will be rendered harmless by the antibodies already present. The antibodies react with the antigen (substances in the bacteria which caused the original antibody formation) and this reaction kills the bacteria. A natural infection in youth leaves a legacy of permanent protection against further attack. Such individuals do not need vaccination. However, those who have avoided natural infection are susceptible to attack in later life which may have more severe and lasting effects. Such individuals require vaccination.

To ascertain the presence of antibodies in the bloodstream and to avoid unnecessary vaccination a test is carried out called the Mantoux test. A small amount of tuberculosis bacterial extract known as tuberculin is injected into the skin. If there is a reaction it will occur in a few days and indicates the presence of antibodies. Only a negative reaction requires further vaccination. It is dangerous to vaccinate people who already have tuberculosis antibodies in the blood.

In England, all schoolchildren between the ages of 10 and 14 are offered a Mantoux test and subsequent B.C.G. vaccination if necessary. B.C.G. may also be given to the newly born babies of tuberculous parents, but the baby must be isolated from its parents for some weeks to give time for the antibodies to develop.

The incidence of tuberculosis in this country has altered considerably since the beginning of the century and to a certain extent has coincided with the availability of B.C.G. vaccination. However, there are many other factors involved. A higher standard of living including better nutrition and an improved standard of housing has probably made as much contribution to the drop in incidence of this disease as has the use of B.C.G., if not more. The main group of people now affected by tuberculosis is old men who live alone and neglect themselves. Some people question the wisdom of continuing to offer B.C.G. to the population and feel that improvement in general standards are sufficient to prevent tuberculosis infection. Others believe that B.C.G. is responsible for the eradication of tuberculosis as a general health hazard in this country.

BED-SORES

Bed-sores occur in people who are enforced—by injury, disease, or infirmity—to sit or lie in one position for a prolonged period without movement. Normally when a person sits or lies he naturally moves his position when he feels pins and needles (paraesthesia) or pain. Both these symptoms indicate untoward pressure on nerves, blood-vessels, and tissues and the consequent necessity for immediate alteration in position. Anyone who is incapable of independent movement while being aware of these symptoms, e.g., because of infirmity in old age or severe illness, or anyone who is unable to perceive these symptoms, e.g., because of spinal injury, multiple sclerosis, or spina bifida, will not respond to the signs of prolonged pressure and this pressure will continue with severe disabling results. The continued pressure prevents blood from reaching the affected area and thus completely removes the oxygen supply to the tissues. Thrombosis or clotting may occur in the affected blood-vessels and there is tissue death. The result is an ulcer or bed-sore.

A large ulcerated area is always prone to infection since the skin, which is the first line of defence against bacterial invasion, is no longer present, and blood-supply to the area is not all that it should be. The infection may spread from the ulcer through the blood-stream to all parts of the body and cause severe generalized infection and death. Factors complicating bed-sores and contributing to the severity include malnutrition and persistent dampness. It is very important that any person exposed to the danger of bedsores should be well nourished and that the skin should be kept well cleansed and dry. Very often those people who are in most danger of developing bed-sores are those who are incontinent of urine. This means that unless great care is taken the skin of the lower part of the body is persistently wet. Anyone who has loss of sensation and movement and who is likely to develop bed-sores should be moved at regular intervals, usually every 2 hours. He or she should be regularly washed, dried, and powdered on those parts exposed to pressure. The person should sit or lie on cushions or sheepskin which allow circulation of air. If possible, the person should raise him or herself frequently. Following surgical procedure or severe illness, the individual should be made to move and walk as soon as possible, and at the first sign of any skin redness, the pressure should be removed from that area. Anyone who has developed bed-sores knows that they take many months to heal. As they most often occur in people who have lost sensation, they are not painful, but can become extensive and deep in a very short space of time.

Alcoholics and drug addicts may develop pressure-sores. Psychiatrists say there is an element of active self-destruction which encourages such people to develop these complications. It may also be so with people who are severely disabled and who may lose the will to live.

It most certainly occurs in the elderly, especially those who have no family or friends and who have no interest in living. Prevention of bed-sores depends on first-class constant nursing attention. In many cases healing of bed-sores requires prolonged hospital treatment and it may be that some people who are disabled feel more secure and can be more dependent in a hospital environment. They may not take all the steps that they should do to prevent development of bed-sores. This is a point to keep in mind when trying to cope with family problems in which repeated hospitalization disrupts family life and causes conflict.

BRONCHIECTASIS

Bronchiectasis is a disease of the lungs which may occur at any age and which refers to the dilatation of the bronchial tubes which are an integral part of the respiratory system. The condition occurs as a complication of other respiratory diseases such as pneumonia, whooping-cough, chronic bronchitis, and asthma, and is often a sequel to a severe attack of measles. It is a chronic condition which continues over many years and gradually reduces respiratory capacity. In many acute lung diseases the bronchial tubes (bronchioles) become plugged with a thick mucus that is produced by the lining of the respiratory passages during any inflammatory condition. This mucus is sticky and difficult to dislodge. Plugs of it completely block portions of the bronchial tubes and cause the formation of dilated sacs. The bronchial tubes lead into the lung tissue which consists of small, thin-walled air sacs, or alveoli. When a bronchial tube becomes cut off by a mucus plug, the alveoli, into which it leads, also dilate and the thin walls of these air sacs break down giving rise to large spaces which can no longer act as efficient oxygen-exchange tissues. These dilated bronchial tubes and large air-sac spaces are filled with pus and other waste substances. Because these areas are stagnant they can easily become infected and abscesses may possibly occur.

Where there is bronchiectasis there is continued bacterial infection. Symptoms include cough, with the production of large amounts of sticky infected mucus, and persistent raised temperature. Blood may also be coughed-up from time to time. These bronchiectatic areas in the lung may heal, but normal tissue is not re-formed and therefore the available amount of lung tissue required for normal air exchange is reduced.

This is a condition which occurs in young children, particularly in association with asthma and as a complication of some of the infectious diseases to which children are particularly prone, e.g., measles and whooping-cough. The timely use of antibiotics may prevent chronic lung damage.

A child suffering with bronchiectasis fails to thrive owing to persistent infection and deficient lung action. He or she spends much time away from school with repeated acute infections of the lungs and, as a consequence of this, fails to develop educationally. This condition tends to be more common in the lower social classes, where large families brought up in poor conditions do not receive efficient medical care in cases of acute childhood ailments. Such children are already living in poor circumstances with insufficient nutrition and lack of cleanliness. Additional frequent school absences and some hospitalization give them a very poor start in life. In other families there is a great deal of overprotection and sheltering of such a frail child, who is not allowed to take part in the activities of his siblings or peers. Parents should be encouraged to allow such a child to participate within his own capabilities. He will know when to stop himself. To completely prevent a child being infected by childhood ailments also means that he will have had to avoid most of the natural childhood pursuits which are so important to the development of any normal well-balanced member of society. Obviously, a child with bronchiectasis is more likely to be affected severely by any superimposed infection. However, the dangers of this must be weighed up very carefully against the even more insidious danger of completely isolating a child from social contact.

Bronchiectasis may be treated by efficient physiotherapy to unblock and move the mucus plugs, by antibiotics, and if necessary by removal of useless damaged lung tissue by surgery. As children with bronchiectasis arrive at puberty and adolescence, their condition tends to improve, although they will always have to take more care than others to protect their lungs from damage.

BRONCHITIS

Bronchitis is known as 'the English disease'. It is particularly prevalent in this country and is thought to be associated with a damp temperate climate and an industrial atmosphere. Acute bronchitis is usually due to bacterial invasion of the lungs and symptoms include a distressing persistent cough, production of large quantities of sputum (phlegm), wheeziness, breathlessness, and a high temperature. The sputum is thick, sticky, and yellow or green in colour. It is sometimes blood-stained. Following treatment with antibiotics symptoms subside and in a healthy person there will be little residual damage within 2–3 weeks.

Chronic bronchitis is the result of repeated attacks of acute bronchitis over a prolonged period. Symptoms are due to permanent, severe lung damage. An individual with chronic bronchitis has a continual cough with sputum, becomes increasingly disabled by breathlessness and wheezing, and may show signs of heart disease. Breathlessness increases in severity until there is difficulty even at rest. Damage to lung tissue results in deficient blood oxygenation. Blood remains a bluish-red colour and imparts a blue tinge to the skin (cyanosis). This is particularly noticeable in the lips, ears, and finger-nails. Lack of oxygenation increases the work load of the heart beyond its capabilities and heart failure gradually develops, aggravating symptoms already present. Death is premature and is usually due to heart failure or overwhelming lung infection reducing the oxygen intake even further. Oxygen deficiency may be so severe in chronic bronchitis that the brain receives insufficient to maintain normal function. Such an individual becomes confused and shows signs of dementia.

The disease is more common in men, particularly those working in industrial conditions. It becomes severe and disabling in middle and later life and is usually aggravated by continued heavy smoking and air pollution. This chronic disease becomes disabling at that period in a man's life when he is also battling with the problems of increasing age and waning powers. The fact that the symptoms may leave him no alternative but to change his job for one with less status and salary, plus the fact that he may have to change his whole way of life, often give rise to family crises and emotional conflict. He may become dependent on his wife for financial support and lose his role as bread-winner. He may need personal help with daily living activities, e.g., dressing and washing. Marital problems may become acute and marital breakdown may occur. Any man disabled by chronic bronchitis should be encouraged to remain independent for as long as possible. The breathlessness is often more distressing to onlookers than to the sufferer. As the disease progresses there will be prolonged periods of superimposed acute infection and more time spent in hospital.

This is a slowly progressive disease with many warning signs. Yearly attacks of acute bronchitis are a good indication of what is in store and it is at this early stage that preventative action should be taken. A relatively young man will have less trouble changing his job and adapting to a new way of life than an older, more disabled individual. It is also important to stress the dangers of continued heavy smoking. It is too late when the man sits breathless in his fireside chair puffing desperately at his only relief—a cigarette.

Chronic bronchitis is not inherited. If it is seen to run in families this is due to the fact that sons often follow fathers into factories and also take up smoking to emulate their parents. It may be that in the future the incidence of bronchitis will increase in women who are tending to smoke more heavily and to work in an industrial atmosphere for longer periods.

CANCER

'Cancer' and 'malignant disease' are terms which refer to a large group of conditions caused by a wide variety of agents. However, the basic abnormality common to all is the replacement of normal tissue cells by abnormal cells which have the power to invade and destroy healthy tissue. These abnormal cells form tumours and also have the facility to travel from the original site of their development to other parts of the body where they invade and destroy and produce secondary tumours in other tissues.

The rate of growth of malignant tumours and the resultant damage depend on a number of factors including age, sex, and the site of the tumour. Cancer cells tend to grow more rapidly in the young. In old age a cancer may be compatible with life for many years. Furthermore, malignant changes in a vital organ are inevitably going to produce fatal results in a short space of time. Some cancers have a propensity for rapid spread to other sites. Others tend to confine themselves to the original site of attack.

In many cases the agent causing the abnormal change is unknown, but in other cases a definite link has been shown between the development of cancer and a predisposing factor. Most causative factors come under three headings: physical, chemical, and viral. Physical factors include X-rays and other radiations. Chemical factors include chemical changes in food induced by cooking processes, the use of fertilizers in agriculture, and the addition of certain substances to foods prior to marketing. Certain chemicals used in industry are also known to cause development of cancer in workers coming into constant contact with them. Some cancers have also been known to develop following invasion of the body by certain viruses. An overriding factor concerned with all these agents is the individual genetic pattern. Exposure to an agent known to induce cancer changes may have no effect on one individual and disastrous effect on another. Some cancers run in families, occurring in the same or similar sites in several members.

General symptoms include loss of weight, tiredness, and loss of appetite. Specific symptoms depend on the site of disease. Later symptoms include general wasting and skin-colour changes. Some cancers can be treated and cured; it depends on the site of the cancer and the nature of the tumour. Some are more malignant than others; some are inaccessible. Treatment methods include radiation, drug therapy, and surgery. The treatment itself may produce severe symptoms, particularly with radiation and drug therapy.

Cancer occurring in a member of a family is always a very distressing experience, particularly if the patient pursues an inexorable path to death. The deterioration is often slow and the person may linger for many months. The problem of communicating about dying is often avoided although many people want to discuss their fears about death. Doctors find dying very difficult to discuss both with relatives and patients as they have not always come to terms with this concept themselves. Death is failure to a doctor and, even though it is an inevitable part of life, such an occurrence is distasteful to a member of the medical profession. The family also finds it difficult and painful to broach the subject and the patient may be isolated, frightened, and extremely lonely at this time. A great deal of support is needed both by family and patient and, if possible, reality must be faced and discussed rationally. Some families cannot cope with a relative with cancer in their own home, particularly as he or she becomes more dependent, and hospital care may be asked for. Treatment and care of the dying patient is a specialized branch of medicine and relatives should be given the utmost help and support.

Many people recover from cancer and a diagnosis of this disease is not a hopeless pronouncement. Continued research improves the outlook and there is every reason to believe that future development will lead to more effective prevention as well as more effective cure.

CARDIAC ARREST

The heart is a vital organ, concerned with supplying the nutritional needs of all the tissues of the body. If the heart ceases its action blood-flow stops, oxygen and other essential substances no longer reach the tissues, and death ensues. Cardiac arrest may occur in a person previously apparently fit and is most often due to coronary thrombosis. It may also occur in individuals with other chronic heart disease. Sometimes drug therapy may cause the heart to stop and this may occur during the administration of a general anaesthetic. But, for whatever reason, it is imperative to start heart action immediately before irreparable damage and death occur.

Muscular movement of the heart may stop completely (asystole) or there may be muscular spasm. In both cases the heart action becomes ineffective. For the layman with no hospital facilities a sharp blow on the chest over the sternum (breast bone) is the first thing that should be done, followed by artificial respiration and external cardiac massage. Mouth-to-mouth breathing is the most effective form of artificial respiration for the lay person, and external heart massage is performed by intermittent regular pressure on the lower end of the sternum (once every second being the most effective rhythm). It is vital to move the patient to hospital as rapidly as possible since the presence of muscle spasm (ventricular fibrillation) requires special treatment. A direct electric current is applied to the chest wall and this usually causes a reversion of heart muscle action to normal rhythm.

Sometimes heart action recovers sufficiently to maintain life with associated irreversible brain damage due to prolonged oxygen deficiency. This may result in paralysis, dementia, or prolonged coma.

CATARACT

The eye is like a camera; light passes through the lens and this normally concentrates the light rays on to the retina to provide an accurate image of the scene upon which the eye is focused. The lens is situated within the eye and is held in place by ligaments. It is composed of fibres which are normally transparent to light.

Cataract is a disease of the lens in which the fibres of the lens become opaque. The fibres may be badly formed at birth giving rise to congenital cataract. Degeneration of the fibres also occurs in advancing age. There are three main types of cataract, known as congenital, acquired, and senile.

Most people have minute lens opacities but in congenital cataract the baby is born with obvious opaque lenses. This may be due to the effect of German measles virus infection prior to birth, maternal malnutrition during pregnancy, or a deficient oxygen supply to the developing baby. Congenital cataract may be partial or complete. Generally speaking, for the purposes of normal daily activities a person with congenital cataract may be said to be blind, although they are often able to distinguish light and dark.

Acquired cataract may be due to many environmental influences such as exposure to ultra-violet light, X-rays, or ultra-sonic radiation. Diabetes may also give rise to lens opacity. However, in most cases of acquired cataract there is no obvious reason, and these may be termed senile cataract, being due to degenerative changes of age. Degeneration of the lens usually starts after the age of 50 and progresses slowly to complete opacity or maturation. It is usually bilateral, but one eye is often affected more severely than the other. The main symptom is visual impairment, which increases in severity until normal daily activity is interrupted and finally light perception is the extent of visual ability.

Treatment of senile cataract is surgical and consists of removal of the lens. This is not performed until the cataract is mature, i.e., the lens is completely opaque. Following surgery sight is corrected by means of suitable spectacles.

CATHETER

A catheter is an instrument which acts as an artificial channel to facilitate the passage of urine, to collect specimens of internal fluids, or to measure physiological functions such as blood-pressure changes at different points in the circulatory system. It is usually flexible and made from rubber or plastic material. However, it can also be rigid and manufactured in steel or other suitable metal.

In connexion with bladder function, catheterization is used preoperatively for complete emptying of the bladder, so preventing damage and facilitating operative technique. Catheterization may also be necessary postoperatively to empty a bladder temporarily paralysed by operative procedure. In cases of persistent bladder paralysis due to disease, accident, or injury a catheter may be inserted as a permanent feature to overcome the problems of incontinence of urine. Urine passing from the bladder into the catheter is collected in a bag which is emptied at suitable intervals. A catheter is also used if an uncontaminated specimen of urine is required for examination.

Catheterization is accompanied by certain hazards. Damage to the urinary apparatus may occur if the instrument is used carelessly or by the inexperienced. A catheter should never be used with force. Introduction of a catheter may also introduce bacteria into the bladder and cause infection.

Catheters are used for investigation of the circulatory system. A very fine polythene catheter introduced into a vein at the elbow may be passed directly into the heart. This manœuvre gives information regarding pressure changes and anatomical abnormalities. Blood specimens can be withdrawn and examined from different areas of the circulatory system normally inaccessible by other methods.

CEREBRAL PALSY

This condition includes a number of abnormalities associated with underlying brain damage sustained before, during, or immediately following birth. The abnormalities are concerned mainly with body movement and posture. Children with cerebral palsy may also have other handicaps including mental subnormality, epilepsy, blindness, deafness, and other physical disabilities.

It is not always possible to define the exact cause of cerebral palsy. Prior to birth, infection in the womb may affect normal brain development, e.g., German measles. Irradiation with X-rays or other radioactive particles may also cause damage. During birth there may be brain damage due to abnormal pressure on the head or oxygen lack. Prolongation of delivery may lead to oxygen deficiency which, if not immediately remedied, causes incurable brain abnormalities. During the immediate postnatal period infections such as meningitis and virus encephalitis may damage the brain and cause cerebral palsy. This condition is also caused in some children by the Rhesus-negative factor. If a woman is Rhesus negative the baby is not necessarily so since the father may be Rhesus positive. Owing to the close association of maternal and foetal blood, antibodies to the Rhesus factor may develop in the mother and pass into the baby. These antibodies cause breakdown of the baby's blood-cells and the breakdown products are deposited in different parts of the body including the brain. This leads to brain damage and cerebral palsy. At the present time it is possible to diagnose this condition prior to birth of the baby and, if immediate transfusion is performed following birth, brain damage can be prevented. However, this treatment is only available in the developed countries of the world.

The major abnormalities are spasticity and rigidity of muscles. All the limbs may be affected and epilepsy is a common accompaniment. Writhing movements known as 'athetosis' may also occur as well as unsteadiness of gait and tremor. The group of children who developed the spastic type of cerebral palsy is thought to comprise those who have suffered brain damage prior to birth. They are often severely mentally retarded. The athetosis type of cerebral palsy is seen in children who have suffered from Rhesus incompatibility and brain injury during birth.

These children are often intelligent and the degree of athetosis is unrelated to the intellectual level.

Children with cerebral palsy may not be diagnosed at birth but they often have feeding difficulties, fail to thrive, and are lethargic. They may show little movement and may be referred to as 'very good' babies. Parents who have children with cerebral palsy require careful and intensive counselling. They also need a great deal of practical help and support. Conflicts between marriage partners are common, with accusations regarding family inheritance coupled with guilt feelings regarding the birth of a severely disabled child. Other children in the family may suffer neglect with all the parental care and attention being given to the disabled child. However, sometimes the child may be completely rejected and neglected and the parents may demand institutional care for their afflicted child.

Cerebral palsy does not preclude ability and talents. Neither does it preclude feelings and desires that any physically able child has. Parents should realize that the child, however severely disabled, must be allowed to grow and mature and to reach his or her maximum potential at all levels. Every child with any disability must learn to be as independent as possible, although in some cases complete independence will never be achieved. There is no cure for cerebral palsy but patience can achieve a great deal. The care and development of a child severely disabled with cerebral palsy require a great deal of patience on the part of parents and often there is a great deal of frustration on the part of both parents and child.

CEREBRAL THROMBOSIS

Blood-vessels supplying brain tissue are subject to degenerative changes due to ageing, known as atherosclerosis. This degeneration makes the inner lining of the blood-vessels rough and irregular and encourages blood-clotting or thrombosis. The brain is very sensitive to alterations in its blood-supply and thrombosis in brain blood-vessels usually leads to permanent disability. If the thrombosis occurs in a blood-vessel supplying that part of the brain concerned with functions vital to life reduction or cessation of blood-flow will cause death. In other cases there will be some degree of recovery, even to the point where there is no evidence of residual damage. Prior to the occurrence of a major thrombosis there are sometimes warning signs—indicating partial occlusion of a blood-vessel—such as pins and needles (paraesthesia) in a limb or speech difficulties.

Residual brain damage depends on the size of the artery affected and the portion of the brain dependent on the affected artery for blood-supply. In the majority of cases there is immediate unconsciousness which may continue until death occurs. In most cases consciousness is recovered after a varying length of time. Other symptoms include paralysis of one or other side of the body, speech problems, visual defects, and emotional disturbances. Left-sided brain damage leads to disability of the right side of the body and vice versa.

Treatment is limited since much of the brain damage is irreversible. There is usually some improvement over the first few weeks, mainly due to the fact that initial irritation and swelling of brain tissue occurring in association with the thrombosis subside. Intelligent and careful nursing is required to avoid bed-sores, pneumonia, and dehydration, all of which can complicate recovery. Physically it is important to avoid deformity in paralysed limbs and active physiotherapy is required from the earliest possible moment. It is also important to start general rehabilitation as soon as possible since morale may be low and motivation poor. If someone who has suffered a stroke sees that he or she has some hope for future life, it is easier to return that person to the community, and everyone with residual disability must be taught to use remaining faculties to the full. In some cases intellect may be affected although this is not usually the biggest problem.

Many people survive for years following a thrombosis or 'stroke' in relatively good health and spirits, but some who survive will always be dependent. Husbands or wives who are left with the burden of caring for a severely disabled marriage partner find themselves faced with physical work at an age when they are finding it increasingly difficult to cope with. Changing beds, toileting, washing, and feeding may all have to be done for the partner who is severely disabled by cerebral thrombosis. Apart from these practical matters there are the emotional problems facing them in day-to-day activities. A wife who has always depended upon her husband will have to take financial responsibilities now and become a leaning-post. Children may find their households disrupted by the arrival of a disabled grandparent. Husbands who have been waited on by wives now find the position reversed. Young married couples with children often find it impossible to accept a parent who can no longer fend for him- or herself. They often refuse to care for a disabled parent who may have to remain in hospital or in a home for the rest of his or her life. The guilt feelings and conflicts arising from this may disrupt family life and even cause marital breakdown.

CHOLESTEROL

Cholesterol is a chemical substance present in the bloodstream. It plays an important part in the transport of fats absorbed into the blood from the digestive tract. It has become particularly important in recent years in relation to heart disease, although the exact role of cholesterol in the development of coronary heart disease and atherosclerosis in general is not yet certain.

Cholesterol is found in all tissues and is present in animal foods normally taken in the daily diet. It is not found in plants. The yolk of an egg contains the highest concentration weight for weight. Butter also contains a considerable amount of cholesterol. Many studies have been done in different areas of the world investigating dietary differences, and it appears from the results of these research projects that diets low in cholesterol are associated with low blood-level concentrations of cholesterol. It also appears that the ingestion of cholesterol alone does not affect blood-levels, but that the type of fat in the diet taken in association with cholesterol has a marked effect on absorption. High blood cholesterol levels are associated with a high incidence of atherosclerosis and coronary heart disease.

A certain amount of cholesterol is lost from the body daily. It passes into the gall-bladder and is excreted with the bile into the intestine. Most of it is reabsorbed but a small amount is lost with the faeces.

CHRISTMAS DISEASE

This is an inherited condition caused by a deficiency in the blood-clotting mechanism. The method by which blood finally clots in response to damage is highly complicated and depends on the presence of a series of chemical substances. If any one of these is missing blood-clotting will be inadequate. In Christmas disease the missing substance is called Christmas factor or factor IX. Because of the inheritance mechanism, the condition is transmitted by the female who does not exhibit the defect. It is the male who suffers the effects of the defect.

Symptoms are similar to those of haemophilia, with spontaneous bleeds, violent and prolonged bleeding in response to minimal injury, joint damage and deformity due to bleeding into joint spaces, and bleeding into the urine. It is most severe before puberty and tends to improve with age.

Blood transfusions are necessary at intervals to restore blood-volume and prevent chronic anaemia.

This condition limits activity, particularly in childhood. This is a very difficult time for parents who want their normal-looking child to grow up normal and yet wish to protect him from injury. School life may be very trying from the point of view of child, teacher, and parent. Any child who is different arouses strong feelings in other children and this makes the growing period a time of trial. Adolescence is beset by problems and sexual relationships will only be complicated by the need for care. However, many people with this condition do lead a normal life. Christmas disease is not a bar to marriage. It is most unwise, however, for there to be children since this is likely to produce females who will carry the disease to their sons. Unless the male with Christmas disease marries a women carrying the defect, boys born to the marriage will not be affected. All these risks should be explained to any couple contemplating marriage. It is difficult to advise people not to have families, but anyone who has suffered from this condition knows from his own experience the very real problems and limitations and must use his own judgement regarding his future reproductive life.

CORONARY HEART DISEASE

Coronary heart disease is due to deficient circulation of blood through the coronary arteries. These arteries supply the heart muscle, which requires oxygen and other substances for adequate nutrition. If the circulation is deficient, the result is pain and functional deficiency. Various abnormalities may reduce coronary circulation. Atherosclerosis may cause hardening of the arteries or there may be a blood-clot (thrombus) blocking the flow of blood. Blood is encouraged to clot by the presence of atherosclerotic damage in the coronary artery walls. A thrombosis may cause partial or complete block in the artery reducing or completely cutting off blood-supply. One or more branches of the coronary artery may be affected and the extent of the heart damage depends on the site of arterial damage. If a large artery is blocked this may destroy heart muscle to the extent that life is not possible.

The disease occurs in middle age and is more common in men. It has become the most important cause of death in this age-group. There have been many hypotheses regarding the increase in incidence of coronary heart disease including stress of modern life, excessive fat intake in the diet, excess consumption of refined sugar, cholesterol, and eggs, intake of soft water, and artificial feeding in infancy. It is possible that some of these may contribute to development of the disease. It may also be possible that the cause of the condition has not yet been discovered.

Symptoms include sudden, severe crushing chest pain, severe breathlessness, nausea, and vomiting. The person affected may lose consciousness and die from cardiac arrest. During the first few days following a coronary attack there is likely to be a further thrombosis and it is essential that the person affected be kept in hospital under constant surveillance (intensive care unit). Other complications include abnormalities of heart-rhythm which may also lead to cardiac arrest and death.

A person surviving the initial attack may well return to leading a normal life, provided that time is allowed for adequate recovery of damaged heart muscle. Individuals who have suffered coronary thrombosis are usually advised to moderate their way of life with regard to eating, drinking, social habits, and employment. There are those who follow this advice and those who do not. As yet there is little proof that those who lead a life of semi-invalidism improve their life expectancy as compared to those who behave as though their hearts have never been affected. Attitude to this condition depends on personality and there are many people who, having suffered severe heart attacks, return to a life no different from that prior to illness. Once advice has been given the decision remains with the individual on whom no one has the right to enforce any limitations. Sometimes marriage partners may prove difficult and act as policemen and watchdogs. This may aggravate the situation since it gives rise to anxiety and stress. Wives must be reassured and given adequate support. They must also be given accurate information. Marital conflict may be more harmful to a person who has suffered a coronary thrombosis than a whisky or a night out on the tiles. Wives are often anxious that sexual activity may have to cease following thrombosis. While it is true that the wife may have to take the active part in the sexual relationship it is not true that this activity must no longer be indulged in. Unfortunately there are those individuals in whom heart muscle is so severely damaged that they can never return to normal life. Conflicts arise due to role reversal and feelings of inadequacy on the part of the man. Professional social workers will be able to give support in this type of situation but the basic medical problem is irreversible at the present time.

CROHN'S DISEASE

Crohn's disease is an inflammation of the lining of the small intestine known as the ileum. The disease is also known as regional ileitis. It is a slowly progressive condition which gradually destroys the inner lining of the ileum. There is no known cause for the development of this disease which usually occurs in the third decade of life. Sometimes the inflammation spreads into the large intestine or colon and even further into the bladder. Sometimes the inflammatory process causes the production of a fistula or artificial connexion between the bowel and the bladder giving rise to chronic kidney and urinary infection.

Symptoms include diarrhoea, loss of weight, and abdominal pain. In some cases the disease appears to cure itself spontaneously. Complications may arise owing to thickening of the bowel wall and narrowing of the intestinal passages. This may give rise to obstruction to the flow of digestive products. Perforation may also occur due to destruction of the bowel wall, leading to haemorrhage into the abdominal cavity and peritonitis. In some cases of Crohn's disease, generalized joint changes occur with rheumatic symptoms of pain and stiffness.

Treatment varies and in many cases is useless. Surgery may be necessary to cope with the complications of obstruction and perforation. Steroid drugs alleviate acute inflammatory episodes of the disease but are not curative. It is important that diet is adjusted to include an adequate amount of potassium since much of this essential substance is lost in the constant diarrhoea. A high-protein diet is considered most suitable.

Many people affected by Crohn's disease lead a reasonably normal life, interrupted by bouts of acute illness. However, in some cases there is a rapid decline and downhill progression and death may occur within a short space of time. This is a condition which occurs in young people and it may cause a great deal of disruption of future plans. It may also prolong the period of parent–child dependence. It is difficult to follow a course of study if this is repeatedly interrupted by acute attacks of ileitis. Social life will inevitably suffer owing to the nature of the disease; continuous diarrhoea makes it impossible to plan any sort of social activity. The disease is not inherited and prospective parents may be reassured on this point. If personal conflicts and problems appear to be aggravating the disease the skills of a professional social worker will be needed to give support and help. It is only natural that a young person suffering from such a chronic debilitating disease should become depressed and need a great deal of support from professional workers and relatives.

CUSHING'S SYNDROME

Cushing's syndrome was first described in 1932, and at that time it was thought to be due to tumours of the pituitary gland. However, recent investigations indicate that most cases of Cushing's syndrome are due to tumours of the adrenal glands with excess production of adrenal hormones (*see* ADDISON'S DISEASE). This condition has also been found to occur in association with cancer of the lung, although this is not common. All the symptoms are due to overproduction of the hormones produced by the adrenal gland, and these include obesity, particularly of the face and body. The skin is pigmented and there are purple markings on many parts of the body. The face may be very hairy and this may be of particular embarrassment in women. Baldness occurs in men and in both sexes the blood-pressure is usually raised. Sexual activity is diminished or may become non-existent with impotence in men and loss of menstruation in women. Hormonal imbalance leads to disturbances in utilization of sugar and to thirst and excess urine production. Psychiatric disturbances may occur. Treatment is by removal of the tumour. Sometimes the tumours invade both adrenal glands and are so extensive that all adrenal tissue has to be removed. This procedure means that although the condition is cured all the hormones normally produced by the adrenal glands, which are essential to life, must be replaced by drug therapy on a permanent basis. Without treatment death will occur prematurely from complications, particularly high blood-pressure.

This disease is unsightly and may cause a great deal of distress, particularly in women. It is frequently undiagnosed until well advanced, since the changes occur over a period of time and are often overlooked by families who are in daily contact with the affected individual. Following treatment, the symptoms usually disappear including the abnormal obesity and pigmentation. Normal life may be resumed providing the person understands the fact that daily tablets are to be a regular and permanent feature.

DEAFNESS

Hearing depends on two factors: the presence of a normal ear and an intact auditory nerve. The ear consists of four parts: a flap or pinna, a channel leading from the exterior to the ear drum, the middle ear, and the inner ear. The middle ear consists of a membrane called the ear drum and three small bones which are connected to each other by joints. The inner ear consists of the cochlea which contains the endings of the auditory nerve.

The external auditory apparatus directs sound waves towards the ear drum. These sound waves cause vibrations of the ear drum which are transmitted via the bones of the middle ear to the cochlea. When the vibrations reach the cochlea they are transmitted along the auditory nerve to the hearing centre in the brain. Here the vibrations are translated into sound. Damage to any part of the hearing apparatus can cause deafness. The external ear may become blocked with secretions or wax preventing sound from travelling to the ear drum. The ear drum is susceptible to infection, particularly in childhood, and it may become rigid and perforated, preventing normal transmission of vibrations. The bones of the middle ear may be affected by arthritis of the joints or by an inherited condition known as osteosclerosis. In these conditions the bones become fused together. The inner ear may be affected by viral or bacterial infection. Some children are born deaf owing to infection in the womb; German measles virus in the unborn child has a particular predilection for the developing ear. With advancing age there may be degeneration of the hearing mechanism and many elderly people suffer with increasing deafness. Damage to the auditory nerve may occur with brain tumours, infections such as meningitis, or atherosclerosis.

Deaf people are not physically repulsive. However, they suffer severely from isolation and loneliness due to problems of communication. Many are underdeveloped intellectually, frustrated in employment, and miserable and isolated socially. Special forms of language have been developed which include finger-spelling, manual communication, and lip-reading. Those who are born deaf have particular problems with language and speech development, conceptualization, and the development of personal relationships. The practical problems of using the telephone, hearing traffic, joining in discussions, and attending the cinema and theatre are often not appreciated by those unaware of what deafness means. Elderly people who lose their hearing may be able to use hearing aids, but sometimes hearing aids are an embarrassment and are abandoned. Old people who are deaf suffer severely from loneliness and isolation. Their families and friends often find it too much trouble to converse with them or include them in conversations.

Isolation in certain situations such as special schools does not help to prepare for integration with the community and often leads to severe problems when the deaf child finally has to take his or her place in a hearing world.

As a deaf child grows towards maturity he or she faces the normal problems of adolescence, marriage, and children, further complicated by inadequate preparation. Deaf people often marry each other and, in many cases, have children who are normal of hearing. This gives rise to many difficulties. Parents tend to use their children as their ears and the children grow to resent this. Although the numbers of severely deaf persons are not large compared to those with other disabilities, this is a serious handicap with far-reaching effects.

It is to be hoped that in the future more thought will be given to providing more adequate community services leading to effective integration into community life.

DIABETES MELLITUS

Diabetes mellitus, colloquially known as sugar diabetes, is a disease resulting from lack of secretion of insulin, a hormone that is secreted by the pancreas and which controls the utilization of sugar by the body. The symptoms that arise are due to an excess of sugar in the blood and to a general disturbance of the utilization of fats, carbohydrates, and proteins by the body. Normally sugar is carried in the blood in the form of glucose. This is derived from carbohydrate in the diet and is carried to all the tissues of the body, providing the energy necessary for survival. There are certain factors which predispose to the development of diabetes. Overeating, particularly of fats, may be responsible for the development of the disease in some people. As overeating is a habit that tends to run in families it is not surprising that several members of one family may have diabetes. It effects a wide age-range of people but is commonly found in those over 40, particularly women. It is not considered that there is any hereditary factor involved.

Many of the presenting symptoms are due to the presence of excess sugar in the blood (hyperglycaemia). Large quantities of dilute urine are produced in an effort to rid the body of sugar. This in turn produces constant thirst in an effort by the body to replace the water lost in the urine. Other symptoms include loss of weight, due to faulty utilization of food; infections, due to the fact that some bacteria thrive in conditions where there is an excess of sugar; failure of vision; and coma, due to the toxic effect of sugar on the brain. Coma may be the first symptom of the diabetic condition. There may be serious secondary complications of the disease. People with diabetes are more prone to suffer from heart disorders and disease of the arteries, pulmonary tuberculosis, cataract, peripheral neuritis, gangrene, and psychosis. These complications are not necessarily avoided even if the diabetes is well controlled by treatment.

Treatment is by replacement therapy in most cases. People suffering from diabetes give themselves daily injections of insulin to control the sugar utilization. In order to make sure that the disease is under good control, urine is tested daily for sugar content by the person himself. In mild cases of diabetes there are available several types of tablets which are able to lower blood-sugar, and which are more acceptable to the patient than self-injection. There are one or two dangers of injection, including local infections and introduction of bacteria into the blood-stream, and people who use insulin must be extremely careful to keep the apparatus sterile, i.e., needles, syringe, etc. There are two types of coma that may be encountered in diabetes. There is the coma due to too much sugar, and that due to too little. If a person taking insulin goes without food, the insulin removes sugar from the blood-stream and there is none to replace it. The brain needs a certain amount of sugar to function effectively, and if this is not available coma ensues. Regular meals have to be taken and should contain very carefully measured quantities of fats, proteins, and carbohydrates. Both kinds of coma should receive immediate hospital attention. Those who have diabetes may be aware of the incipient onset of coma and can take the necessary precautions in some cases. The immediate ingestion of sugar may avert insulin coma.

Those with diabetes can lead perfectly normal lives provided that they observe certain rules. Extra effort usually requires extra insulin, particularly pregnancy and operative procedures. Pregnancy in a diabetic woman often ends in disaster since many babies born to a diabetic mother die soon after birth. This is not to say that a woman with diabetes should not have children, but she will need very careful supervision during pregnancy. An acute infection in a diabetic must be treated with great respect and immediate expert medical advice should be sought. As far as working life is concerned, there need be no great upheaval as long as colleagues are aware of the fact that the person has diabetes and that they know a little bit about the condition. They may be able to spot the incipient development of coma before the individual himself. Excess irritability often indicates that the person is not as well controlled as usual as far as his diabetes is concerned, and he should be advised to consult his doctor.

DOWN'S SYNDROME

Mongolism or Down's syndrome is due to a genetic defect involving the chromosomes. Normally every person has forty-six chromosomes in each body cell, but a mongol has forty-seven. This chromosomal abnormality gives rise to a low-grade mental defective with very characteristic facial configuration including slant eyes, flat nasal bridge, small skull, protruding tongue, and slender neck. The tongue becomes deeply fissured from constant sucking; the hands are distinctive with short fingers and only one palmar crease; the hair is straight. Other abnormalities are also associated, including congenital heart disease, obstruction in parts of the digestive tract, particularly in the oesophagus and the anus, and deafness.

Individuals affected by mongolism are particularly susceptible to respiratory-tract infections and until the development of antibiotics very few survived to adulthood. However, they now live to middle age and beyond. Mongols are usually good-natured and learn to walk, talk, feed themselves, and do simple tasks. Some can be employed provided that the job is easy and repetitive and that the employer is agreeable to employing them. When very young they may appear to be developing normally but retardation becomes obvious as the child matures chronologically. Parents of mongol children often exhibit guilt feelings and emotions associated with giving birth to an abnormal child, but as the child develops and begins to communicate he or she is usually accepted by the other children and may present few problems, at least until adulthood.

Mongol children usually attend training centres for mentally defective children. This helps to relieve the mother from having the child in the house permanently and also helps to socialize the child. Many parents worry about having further children following the birth of a mongol. In a young mother it may well be inadvisable to have another child, and the genetic patterns of the parents should be fully investigated. In an older mother a mongol child is usually the last of her pregnancies.

It is not always possible to diagnose mongolism at birth and it is very hard to tell parents that their child is a mental defective after a few weeks when close bonds have been formed. Sometimes it may be 3–6 months before one can say with accuracy that the baby is a mongol. It is vital that the parents be told about their child in a gentle and careful manner. They should understand the facts and be given accurate information. Even when parents are told, they often find it difficult to equate their apparently normal baby with their experience of a mongol child. It may take many months before a mother will accept the facts. Experienced counselling is of paramount importance, as parents are usually most anxious about future prospects.

DRUG ADDICTION

Drugs are taken for a variety of medical reasons. Normally when the medical reason no longer exists the drugs are no longer of use and they are no longer administered. However, there are those people who take drugs for other than medical needs. These people become unable to continue normal daily activity without drugs and are called drug addicts.

Drug addiction has been common in the United States of America for some years and is becoming an increasing problem in this country. The relatively free prescription of such drugs as barbiturates and amphetamines for such conditions as insomnia and anxiety leads to a large-scale use of these by people, some of whom eventually become addicts. Teenagers are particularly vulnerable to the use of drugs, and the 'permissive society' attitudes are in some measure responsible for the increase in numbers of teenagers who become drug addicts.

There are many reasons for the development of drug addiction. These may be grouped under social, psychological, and physical headings. Socially, some young people are easily led and will try anything once. Others want to be part of the scene and do not want to be left out. As mentioned previously, it is easy to obtain drugs which give a pleasant effect and which leave the person wanting further experience of the drug. Psychologically, some people need a prop. Some get their props from alcohol, some start smoking, and others take drugs. Some are unable to accept and cope with life's difficulties. Others seek new experiences and pleasures. Some are severely disturbed and need psychiatric help. From a physical point of view, some people who have been given drugs to relieve pain find that they cannot do without these drugs. It is also thought that certain personalities require different types of drugs, depending on the chemical make-up of the individual. Some require heightening of the emotions, others want to deaden feelings.

Some drugs are habit forming rather than addictive. Withdrawal of such drugs is unpleasant but does not give rise to physical symptoms. These include the amphetamines, cocaine, L.S.D., and marihuana. Others are addictive and withdrawal gives rise to severe physical symptoms. These include the opiates such as morphine and heroin.

Diagnosis of drug addiction may be difficult. Addicts do not usually wish to reveal their weakness. However, morphine and heroin addicts will show marks of needles, particularly on their forearms. Those who take morphine have permanently constricted pupils. Oral addiction is more difficult to uncover.

Treatment is difficult since it relies on the co-operation of the patient. Confidence must be gained and the drug stopped. Withdrawal symptoms can be avoided by heavy sedation. These symptoms include watering of the eyes and nose, sneezing, shivering, severe abdominal pain, vomiting, and nausea. Following withdrawal an intensive rehabilitation programme must be followed. It is more than likely that a return to the original environment will lead to breakdown. The person under treatment should stay in a sheltered environment to regain confidence and feel some sense of security. If necessary his whole life should alter, including residence, job, and social life. He must also have the support of relatives and friends if possible.

The expectation of life for an addict is not good. He is more likely to succumb to severe infection due to the use of dirty hypodermic needles and malnutrition. Even those on oral drugs are more likely to be severely affected by any infection contracted.

Addicts are sick people, not criminals. However, they do like to convert other people to the cause and they often tend to frequent places where the young and impressionable may be seduced. In this way the addict may be said to be behaving anti-socially. Addicts may also commit criminal acts in order to obtain finances to purchase drugs. They are often more likely to end up in police courts than in hospitals.

The problem of drug addiction is closely associated with parental attitudes and parent–child relationships. The breakdown of family groups, the freedom and affluence of the young, plus the lack of purpose that may exist and the threat of war and destruction, all serve to undermine the confidence and security of modern youth. The whole problem needs consideration on a much wider basis and drug addiction must be considered as a major symptom of social disintegration.

ECZEMA

Eczema is a skin disorder caused by a wide variety of agents. It is often associated in childhood with asthma. The condition may be inherited and can often be seen in other members of the family. It is aggravated by emotional disturbances but it can also cause conflict and stress by its nature. It is unsightly and irritable and causes lack of sleep.

It first appears on parts of the body exposed to the agents causing it, but it can spread to other parts. Eczema only occurs in those people who are predisposed to it; agents causing eczema in susceptible people do not affect those who are not susceptible.

Eczema often occurs in fat people or in areas of varicose veins where blood-flow is slowed down. Fair skins tend to be more prone to development of eczema.

Symptoms include itchiness, redness, dryness, and scaliness of the skin. Sometimes the eczema becomes infected due to scratching and pus forms, with associated rise in temperature and other signs of infection.

Eczema–asthma sufferers usually start at about 6 months of age and the eczema appears mainly on the face and the limb flexures. A proportion of these people develop hay fever in adolescence, others develop arthritis.

In treating eczema the cause should be found. Local treatments to relieve irritation include steroid ointments which relieve inflammation. Drugs may be needed to give the patient some rest.

Eczema causes many problems, particularly in schoolchildren. Because of the unsightliness of the condition children may be ostracized and have no friends. They may have long periods out of school when the condition becomes severe and the associated asthma may also cause school absences. Although the condition seems to clear up as the child matures, the emotional damage has been done and the child can remain isolated, shy, and lonely. In later life the skin sensitivity may cause some practical problems. Washing powders and water often aggravate any eczematous tendency and young housewives may find themselves somewhat limited by repeated attacks of eczema on their hands. Once again one must consider the inheritance factor when advising parents on the possibilities of affected children. The predisposition to develop eczema is inherited, but not every child who is born to affected parents will be affected. Eczema and asthma can cause a great deal of misery in an infant and child, and anyone who has suffered the condition should think twice about passing on the inheritance to another human being.

EMPHYSEMA

Emphysema is a chronic condition affecting the lungs. Lungs consist of air sacs which have very thin walls. Blood-vessels run in close proximity to the air sacs and there is an exchange of gases between the blood-vessels and the air sacs, made possible due to the fact that the walls separating air sac and blood are thin enough to be permeable to gases. It is in the lungs that oxygen passes into the blood and carbon dioxide is returned to the external environment. Obstruction to respiration occurs in chronic bronchitis and asthma. The lungs are required to work against this obstruction and, as a consequence, the air sacs dilate. The walls between the air sacs rupture and large cavities or bullae are formed. This condition is known as emphysema.

Emphysema adds to respiratory embarrassment in chronic lung disease by further damaging lung tissue.

Symptoms include breathlessness and blood-stained sputum. The skin is blue-tinged (cyanosis) owing to reduction of oxygen content in the blood. Heart failure may also develop. The lung changes are irreversible; however, the symptoms may be alleviated by treating the primary disease. Exercises may also help to improve the capacity of the chest. Climate is important and any chronic chest condition is helped by a warm, dry atmosphere. Chronic bronchitis is inevitably accompanied by some degree of emphysema, which is a progressive complication. Air sacs continue to dilate and their walls to rupture with the development of bullae until the amount of normal lung tissue remaining is inadequate to support life.

ENURESIS

Enuresis refers to the failure of development in voluntary control of emptying of the bladder at an age when most children are able to control this function adequately.

Voluntary control of the bladder by day is normally established by the age of 2 although night control may not be fully developed until the age of 3. To a certain extent the development of control depends on training. If a family does not expect a child to be dry, such a child will not feel the necessity to develop this habit. A child who remains in nappies over a certain age does not receive the correct stimulation to development of bladder control. Any child who has learnt to empty his or her bladder when necessary may temporarily lose this facility through illness or emotional upset. One of the commonest reasons for development of enuresis is the arrival of a new baby and the apparent rejection of the older child. It is more common for children to continue to wet the bed at night although they may be in full control during the daytime.

Enuresis is a symptom of abnormal functioning and may be due to underlying organic disease. Any child suffering from enuresis must receive a thorough physical examination. Spina bifida and epilepsy are both causes of enuresis. Some children have congenital malformations of the urinary tract which prevent voluntary bladder control. Any acute or chronic illness may give rise to bed-wetting.

However, the main cause of enuresis is emotional disturbance and when organic disease has been excluded the child and his family must be considered in the light of emotional development. There may be parental conflict and marital disharmony. The child may suffer from insecurity. His parents may be divorced and may use him to satisfy their own emotional needs. More attention may be lavished on a younger child who may be more attractive or who may require more attention owing to disability. An overprotective mother may cause the child to develop enuresis.

Most enuretic children are heavy sleepers and are not disturbed by a wet bed. Punishment creates further emotional disturbance and the situation becomes a vicious circle.

Various treatments have been devised to cure enuresis. Obviously, any organic lesion should be treated and emotional disturbance investigated. There are various drugs which may help by preventing too deep a sleep. There is also an electric device which involves a bell ringing when bed-wetting occurs. Used over a period of time the child may be conditioned to wake before the bell rings, i.e., before wetting occurs.

There is a tendency for enuresis to cure itself. However, it can cause a great deal of worry to the child and to his parents which tends to perpetuate the defect. The problem of smell in a child who is continually wet may cause his isolation at school. Difficulties with bed-wetting may lead to exclusion from holidays and outings. Careful handling of this condition is essential and the problem is not solved by keeping the child in nappies. If parents can be made to understand that this is merely a temporary failure in the natural process occurring in the child and to treat the condition with common sense it will tend to disappear more rapidly than if treated with undue seriousness and with disapproval.

EPILEPSY

Epilepsy is not a disease; it is a group of symptoms indicative of abnormal functioning of the brain tissue. There are many variations in the symptoms in different individuals. The main symptoms include warning signs (the aura), loss of consciousness, muscle spasm, jerking involuntary limb movements, and involuntary bladder and bowel evacuation. There are two main types of epilepsy: idiopathic and symptomatic. Epilepsy is called idiopathic when there is no obvious underlying cause. This type of epilepsy usually begins in childhood or adolescence and may be found in other members of the family. Symptomatic epilepsy refers to epilepsy due to brain disease such as tumour, injury, or high blood-pressure. It usually occurs in adulthood and may be associated with other signs and symptoms of brain disease.

Epilepsy may take one of several common forms, which are major fits or grand mal, minor fits or petit mal, and focal fits or Jacksonian epilepsy. In grand mal there is a brief aura lasting several seconds which may be just a feeling, or be associated with one of the senses, such as a hallucination, a smell, or a sound. This is quickly followed by loss of consciousness, involuntary limb and body movements, bladder and bowel action. The third stage of the fit is a coma when the body returns to normal. The actual fit is followed by a period of confusion and drowsiness. The whole procedure may last from a few minutes to several hours including the after-effects. These types of fits are not usually a frequent occurrence. They are common in idiopathic epilepsy and are often triggered off at a particular time in the day, or night, or by certain occurrences such as emotional stress or menstruation.

The minor fits are common in the idiopathic epilepsy of children. These are brief lapses of consciousness without coma, which appear as a momentary lack of concentration. The individual is unaware of these and carries on normally when they pass. They may occur many times in a day.

Jacksonian fits are associated with brain damage due to growing tumours or severe brain damage. There is always an aura, varying in each individual depending on which part of the brain is affected. Once again it may be a particular smell or noise. A phenomenon associated with Jacksonian fits is the *déjà vu* when the person feels as though he has been before in the exact situation in which he finds himself. This aura is followed by involuntary movement of a remote part of the body, such as a toe, and this movement spreads to extend over the whole of the affected side. There is no loss of consciousness and the whole fit lasts only a few seconds.

Status epilepticus is a condition where one fit follows another without a break and which often occurs with sudden drug withdrawal. It may be fatal due to exhaustion and irreversible high temperature.

Epilepsy can be controlled by drugs if it is idiopathic. Drugs can alleviate symptomatic epilepsy but the underlying cause should be the primary aspect of treatment. It is idiopathic epilepsy which gives rise to the majority of problems associated with epilepsy. The public are frightened of this condition and there are strong primitive remnants of the old attitudes towards a 'disease of the devil'. Epileptics are restricted from leading a normal life even if well controlled. Employment is difficult, particularly for manual workers. Individual employers do not want to risk the threat of industrial accident and compensation. Other employees do not want to work with an epileptic. Professions such as medicine are barred to those who have epilepsy, even though they have normal intellect and enthusiasm.

Epileptics may not drive until free from daytime fits for 3 years. They are restricted in their activities at school, including swimming and games. School is a particularly difficult time for children with epilepsy. Exclusion always makes children feel different and out of things, and other children tend to exclude them from other activities. They are lonely children who are overprotected at home and rejected at school. Often, medication to prevent fits makes them dopey and they appear to be slow and stupid at scholastic efforts; and, in any case, many lose much schooling from absences due to illness and hospitalization. It is important that the public should be educated about the nature of epilepsy. Epilepsy may be inherited and this should be kept in mind when counselling prospective parents.

FLATULENCE

This annoying condition is due to swallowing of air. The passage of air via the mouth or the bowel is known as eructation. People who suffer with flatulence experience a sensation of fullness and distension with abdominal discomfort. Relief is achieved by eructation but is usually followed by further swallowing of air and further symptoms. Air-swallowing occurs during meals which are hurried and hastily chewed. The air may pass into the small intestine and give rise to embarrassing noises (borborygmi).

Flatulence is not usually a symptom of disease although it may be associated with abnormalities of the digestive tract. It can occur in chronic gall-bladder disease and cancer of the stomach. Gall-bladder flatulence is due to swallowed air and abnormal movement of the stomach wall.

Flatulence can be improved by eating slowly and chewing well and by resting for a period after meals. It is said that a pipe or cigarette holder in the mouth after a meal will prevent further air-swallowing, but the major damage is done during a meal (when it is not usual to smoke and eat at the same time).

This can be a most embarrassing abnormality although everyone suffers with it from time to time. It is easier to control eructation via the mouth. Bowel eructation often occurs involuntarily. It is not a condition likely to be the major problem in any case. If it is, the social worker may be dealing with serious disease or a neurosis and medical aid should be sought rapidly.

FRIEDREICH'S ATAXIA

Friedreich's ataxia, also known as hereditary spinal ataxia, is an inherited chronic progressive disease affecting the nervous system. It may occur in several members of the same family or in several generations. The first symptoms of the disease usually appear between the ages of 5 and 15, although the onset may be delayed until adulthood. The condition appears equally in boys and girls.

The degenerative disease process takes place in those parts of the spinal cord responsible for the control of muscle behaviour. The main symptoms of the illness are due to a loss of muscle control which results in defective balance and incoordination of movement. Other effects of this degeneration include loss of power in limbs, particularly in the feet and the legs, with resultant contractures and deformities. Imbalance of muscle control also leads to spinal deformities, and a tremor which is most marked when the limbs are engaged in purposeful activity. Slurred speech may occur and is due to disordered action of the tongue muscle and other organs related to speech production.

Later effects of the disease are due to degeneration of brain tissue and include mental deterioration. The condition is progressive; the person affected usually ends his or her days confined to a wheel-chair, if not bed-bound. This enforced immobility gives rise to the secondary complications of bed-sores and pneumonia, which are common in all conditions where the affected is unable to move freely. Premature death occurs in most cases of Friedreich's ataxia between 10 and 15 years after the onset of the disease. However, occasionally there may be an arrest of symptoms and the person may live a normal life-span. There is no specific treatment, but physiotherapy and regular exercise will prevent crippling deformities.

There is no reason why a person with this condition should not be considered for training for some kind of occupation, since he or she may well be fit to work for several years. Of necessity the work considered should be of a sedentary nature. It is difficult to advise people about marriage and having children. But as the disease has a strong hereditary factor much thought should be given to the problem before a person who has the disease takes on the role of parent. Even if the child is perfectly normal the fact that he is going to be deprived of one parent from a relatively early age is something that should be taken into serious consideration.

GALL-STONES

Gall-stones are formed in the gall-bladder. This is a small sac connected to the liver by channels called bile-ducts. The gall-bladder stores bile. Bile consists of bile-salts and bile-pigments, both of which are manufactured by the liver. Bile-salts are important in the processes of fat digestion and help to emulsify fats in the small intestine so that they can be absorbed easily. Bile-pigments are breakdown products from old red blood-cells. These are useless and are removed from the body by being excreted with the bile in the intestine. Bile-pigments are responsible for the distinctive yellowish-green colour of the bile. The gall-bladder stores the bile until it is required. When the contents of the stomach enter the small intestine this stimulates contraction of the gall-bladder and bile enters the small intestine through connecting channels between the two organs. Bile can then mix with the intestinal contents.

Gall-stones consist of calcium, cholesterol, and bile-pigments in combination. There may be many of them inside the gall-bladder and, if numerous, they give rise to symptoms causing a great deal of distress. They are more common in women and are often associated with bacterial infection. The gall-bladder may become abnormally enlarged and be felt on examination. It is normally situated behind the liver and is not palpable.

Many of the symptoms may be due to obstruction of bile outflow by stones impacted in the ducts. These induce severe pain, jaundice, and infection. The pain is due to muscular spasm as the gall-bladder tries to expel the stones. Jaundice is due to back-flow of bile-pigments which overflow into the blood-stream and tissues. Bacterial infection often occurs where there is stagnation of body fluids. Infection in the gall-bladder will give rise to various symptoms including a high temperature, nausea, and vomiting, as well as pain and jaundice.

This condition may be associated with abnormal diets such as too much fat intake. It is important to alter diet in this disease but the only effective cure is surgery.

GASTRIC ULCER

Gastric ulcers affect the lining of the stomach wall. There are also similar ulcers affecting the lining of the next part of the digestive tract, the duodenum. Both gastric and duodenal ulcers are also known as peptic ulcers. Over recent years duodenal ulcers have become more common than gastric ulcers, the reason for this being obscure. Gastric ulcers affect those parts of the stomach wall bathed in gastric juice. This fluid contains a weak acid and other substances which break down food into simpler substances that can be absorbed into the blood-stream.

There is a familial incidence of gastric ulcers and these tend to occur in the same site, indicating an inherited weakness. Many causes have been cited for the development of ulceration, including worry and stress. Emotion has a great effect on stomach or gastric juice. However, there is no absolute evidence that the worrying personality has more chance of developing ulcers. It is also possible that highly spiced food may have an irritating effect on the stomach lining. Aspirin taken on an empty stomach often precipitates the development of ulcers in the stomach and other drugs may have the same effect. Bad teeth, alcohol, tobacco, and irregular meals have all been incriminated, but it is more likely that these agents merely aggravate a condition already present.

The actual ulcer consists of damage to the stomach lining and symptoms include abdominal pain relieved by food, nausea, and vomiting. Complications include perforation of the stomach wall, with release of stomach contents into the abdominal cavity leading to peritonitis and death if not treated. Other complications include development of cancer at the ulcer site, massive haemorrhage due to erosion of a blood-vessel, and obstruction to passage of food due to inflammation and narrowing of the stomach.

The treatment of gastric ulcer varies depending on the severity of symptoms and the acuteness of onset and the precipitating cause. Most cases can be treated successfully by bed-rest, diet, and alkali drugs to relieve the acidity. Small meals at frequent intervals help the healing process considerably. Surgery is only resorted to in certain circumstances including failure of medical treatment, possibility of cancer, and complications such as perforation or haemorrhage.

People who suffer with gastric ulcers tend to be in pain for a great deal of time. This makes them bad-tempered and difficult to live with. They have problems with eating and drinking and this limits their social life considerably. The so-called typical ulcer appearance, of a haggard, drawn, lined face, is the result of many years of coping with pain and discomfort. Marital conflict may arise due to continued irritability of the suffering marriage partner, who may not be able to fulfil his or her expected role in the marital relationship.

GLAUCOMA

The term 'glaucoma' refers to raised pressure within the eye. This raised pressure may be due to excess fluid within the eye or to an artificial block to outflow channels. There are two major types which are known as congestive and simple.

Congestive glaucoma occurs as an acute condition with severe headache and pain in the eye. There is impairment of vision and the development of 'halo formation'—a subjective sensation where lights are seen to have haloes surrounding them. Normally there is fluid within the eye responsible for nutrition and removal of waste products. In congestive glaucoma drainage of fluid is prevented by a block in the drainage channels. The attack of glaucoma usually starts at night and in the dark. The pupil dilates in darkness and this further decreases the size of the drainage exit. Nausea and vomiting may accompany the other symptoms.

The condition may be treated medically by constricting the pupil, by removing excess fluid, and by sedation. Surgically it is possible to enlarge the drainage channels.

Simple glaucoma occurs insidiously and there is a gradual diminution of fields of vision which may go unnoticed by the patient until vision is grossly disturbed. There is usually no pain or other acute symptom. The cause is considered to be due to changes in blood-vessels due to atherosclerosis, with resultant decrease in blood-supply to eye tissues and damage to these tissues due to malnutrition.

Both these types of glaucoma are considered to be inherited in a large proportion of cases and are also associated with conscientious, worrying types of personalities.

Early diagnosis of simple glaucoma is essential to prevent damage which is irreversible once it occurs. Lack of symptoms makes this difficult and general population screening would perform a useful function in early detection of this condition. Treatment is to trace the cause which will include generalized treatment of atherosclerosis. Improving drainage by constriction of the pupil and removing excess fluid by drug therapy are also of use in attenuating the condition.

Glaucoma is the commonest cause of blindness in older age-groups.

GONORRHOEA

Gonorrhoea is one of a group of diseases known as 'venereal'. This term refers to the fact that in the majority of cases the infection is passed on by sexual contact. Gonorrhoea is caused by a bacterium and a person may be infected for several days before symptoms appear. It is during this period of incubation that the person is most liable to spread infection to others.

Several days after infection occurs there is production of a thick, yellow, purulent discharge from the genital passages. The complications of this acute bacterial inflammation may cause lasting and distressing disability. In the male, inflammation may cause narrowing of the genital passage or urethra and may cause great difficulty in the passage of urine in later years. Obstruction to urinary flow causes damage and deterioration of kidney tissue. In the female the discharge may not be so obvious, which gives the added danger that such an infected woman may continue to have intercourse while not realizing that she has contracted gonorrhoea. The later complications of the inflammatory process in women include chronic inflammation of the womb (uterus) and the Fallopian tubes, leading to sterility and chronic ill health. A woman infected during pregnancy is a particular danger to her unborn child since, during passage of the baby along the birth canal, infection of the eyes may lead to blindness in the infant.

Gonorrhoea is easily curable with the use of penicillin. It is also important that all sexual contacts of the infected person should be traced and treated. This may cause serious marital difficulties since an innocent marriage partner may be totally unaware of the extramarital activities of a spouse until informed that he or she has a venereal disease.

Although the basic cause of the infection is a bacterium, there are associated important social causes. The disease is prevalent in low socio-economic groups where overcrowding, poverty, and human degradation lead to prostitution and infection. It also becomes widespread during wars when soldiers seek solace with prostitutes and promiscuous women. Affluent societies often have upsurges of gonorrhoea due to disintegration of parental control, disintegration of family life, and the long latent period between sexual maturity and the age of marriage. Sexual freedom and a 'permissive' society lead to experimentation and free expression of the young in the field of sexual activity. A high illegitimacy rate is usually associated with a high rate of venereal infection. Marriage conflict is common in affluent civilization due to the higher expectations of each partner. Divorce is easily obtainable.

All these factors encourage the spread of venereal disease and, although it is relatively easy to cure gonorrohoea, the basic problems of an affluent, sophisticated society are often insoluble.

HAEMOPHILIA

This disease is due to an inherited defect in the mechanism of blood-coagulation. It is transmitted through the female but exhibited only in the male (with rare exceptions). One of the substances involved in clotting is known as factor VII and it is a deficiency of this which causes the symptoms.

Symptoms begin in infancy and become less severe after puberty although they continue throughout life. Bleeding may occur spontaneously or from very slight injuries, with persistent oozing for many hours. Bruising may be extensive and bleeding is particularly common into joints and the urine. Complications include severe anaemia and damage to joints leading to osteo-arthritis.

Treatment is by blood transfusions and the prevention of injuries and joint damage should be treated with extreme care to avoid disability.

The problems of this disease are those associated with the normal life activities of small children. A child with haemophilia cannot be allowed to take part in the rough and tumble of nursery and school life without a great deal of damage and perhaps even risk to life. Any child who feels and looks normal and yet is excluded from the activities that are his right must suffer severe psychological trauma in the formative and growing years. Parents are right to be anxious and yet they should try to permit freedom as far as they are able. It is very difficult to achieve the correct balance. The school should know about the disability and understand the severity of the condition. In this way they may well be able to include the child in many activities provided they have the co-operation and understanding of the other children. As the child grows up he faces the problem of puberty and adolescence. He wants to lead a normal teenage life but this is often difficult, if not impossible. He will need a great deal of help to come to terms with his prospects and it may be a long and difficult task. The problem of reproducing is one which occurs more often these days since haemophiliacs now survive to reproductive and marriageable age. It is most unwise for a male haemophiliac sufferer to have children since he may pass on the inherited tendency to his daughters who, in their turn, may have sons that will be affected. Women of a haemophilic family should be very carefully investigated before they have children since, although they do not exhibit the symptoms, they may well be carrying the disease and will pass it to any sons they may have. It is difficult to advise people against having children but it is even more difficult—from both a physical and emotional point of view—to rear a child with haemophilia.

HAY FEVER

Hay fever is a seasonal affliction caused by sensitization of the upper respiratory tract to grass pollens which are carried in the atmosphere between May and July each year. The conjunctivae are also affected. Those people who become sensitized often exhibit other allergic phenomena such as eczema and asthma. Asthma often develops as a consequence of persistent recurrent hay fever.

Symptoms include sneezing, coughing, and irritation, watering of the eyes, and nasal congestion. All these symptoms occur in varying degrees of severity. The onset of hay fever may occur at any age but most commonly originates in adolescence. It often improves with ageing, although it may persist for many years. Treatment is difficult. It is possible to produce a state of hyposensitization by a series of injections of pollen extract. However, this must be done some time before the start of the pollen season and may need to be repeated each year. Antihistamine tablets may relieve symptoms but have side-effects which may affect school and work. They tend to induce drowsiness and driving a car is ill-advised if antihistamine drugs are being prescribed.

The symptoms of hay fever can be most distressing and affect the daily life of the individual to a considerable extent. The persistent sneezing and general nasal obstruction can lead to depression and instability and prevent concentration on the task in hand. Schooling may suffer because of lack of concentration and headache. Pressure of work may be made intolerable by the addition of hay-fever symptoms. While in the main the disease has nuisance value rather than serious implications, the persistent presence of upper respiratory-tract symptoms may have a great deal of influence on the individual in affecting his or her way of life. Anyone who has hay fever and is sensitive to pollen is potentially liable to develop sensitivity to other things and should beware of contact with objects notorious for causing sensitivity reactions, e.g., plants such as primulas, and certain foods such as crab and strawberries.

THE HEART

The heart is a muscular organ concerned with pumping blood around the body. It consists of four chambers: a left auricle and ventricle, and a right auricle and ventricle. The right auricle receives blood from the body tissues through the vena cava vein and passes it to the right ventricle. From the right ventricle blood passes to the lungs through pulmonary arteries, comes into close contact with air in lung tissue, absorbs oxygen, and is returned to the left auricle via the pulmonary veins. From the left auricle blood passes into the left ventricle and thence to all parts of the body through the artery known as the aorta, thus supplying body needs.

There is a system of valves which prevents back-flow during the powerful heart contractions. The mitral valve separates the left auricle and ventricle; the tricuspid valve separates the right auricle and ventricle. There is also a valve between the aorta and the left ventricle and between the pulmonary artery and the right ventricle.

The heart muscle has an intrinsic rhythm of contraction and relaxation which is placed at the sinus, a small area of heart tissue which acts as the control. The pacemaker signals are transmitted through a specialized bundle of heart-muscle fibres known as the bundle of His. The heart rhythm is also affected via the central nervous system through nerve-fibres supplying heart muscles.

The blood supplies body tissues with oxygen and removes carbon dioxide which is a waste product of human metabolism. Food which is broken down to glucose reacts with oxygen brought by the blood-stream to provide energy for all body activities and carbon dioxide is also produced in this reaction.

The heart muscle is supplied by the coronary arteries since the muscle requires oxygen for energy just as much as any other tissue. If any part of the heart muscle does not receive oxygen it dies and can no longer take part in the total heart action. If too much heart muscle is killed by lack of oxygen the heart can no longer function. The coronary arteries form a network of branches supplying all parts of the heart. There is a left branch supplying the left side of the heart and a right branch supplying the right side, with some interconnecting branches. The work of the left side is much harder since blood has to be pumped with more force to reach the farthest parts of the body. Thus the blood-supply to the left side is greater. There are also branches of the coronary arteries which are not normally used but which can be utilized if other parts of the coronary artery system are put out of action.

HODGKIN'S DISEASE

This is a disease affecting the lymph-glands, spleen, and liver. The normal tissues of these organs become replaced by abnormal cells and normal function is lost. The lymph-glands and spleen produce white blood-cells which are responsible for body defence against bacteria and other toxic agents. Defence mechanisms include ingestion of bacteria and other products by the white cells. White cells are also responsible for the production of antibodies, another form of defence. In Hodgkin's disease there is a gradual reduction in the number of white cells in the body with resultant anaemia. Death usually occurs from massive infection due to lack of body-defence mechanisms. The disease is a type of cancer. It affects young people and is common in males. Abnormal tissue can spread from lymph-glands to other organs and can be found in lung tissue and in bone-marrow. If deposits of abnormal cells occur in the lungs symptoms associated with abnormal lung function may be the first indication of the disease, i.e., breathlessness and coughing. Other symptoms include tiredness, a raised temperature, and the presence of large, painless, rubbery glands. Occasionally a secondary deposit in the spine may cause paraplegia.

Various treatments include surgery to remove glands, X-rays, drug therapy, and blood transfusions. A person may survive for up to 10–12 years or may die several weeks after onset. The emotional and psychological problems associated with this disease are those associated with any cancer but are complicated by the youth of the person and by the uncertainty of the prognosis. Treatment is time-consuming and often has side-effects more unpleasant than the disease itself. Remission can occur following treatment, raising hopes of the patient, often unrealistically. If the patient can manage to continue his work and his home life he should be encouraged to do so, since lack of purpose will add further to the psychological problems encountered. Some sufferers will not be aware that they have such a serious illness, but their spouses and families will know and may require help to cope with this knowledge. Some individuals may require a great deal of support as they try to cope with the idea of premature death.

HORMONES

Hormones are essential chemical substances produced by various glands in the body and which pass directly into the blood-stream. They are required in very small quantities but are necessary for the control of essential body function. These substances are carried in the bloodstream to the whole body and act on various tissues. Hormonal activities are concerned with the control of metabolic processes, sexual function, reproductive function, growth and tissue replacement, and central nervous system function.

The pituitary gland (*see* PITUITARY GLAND) is known as the master gland and produces various hormones which affect the other glands producing hormones, i.e., the adrenal gland, thyroid, ovaries, testicles, parathyroid gland, and the pancreas. If the pituitary hormones fail then the glands which they control also fail to produce hormones.

HUNTINGTON'S CHOREA

This is a rare disease which is due to an inherited defect. It occurs in one or more members of the same family in each generation. The basic defect is a degeneration of certain areas of the brain giving rise to abnormal involuntary movements, deterioration of speech, alterations in personality, loss of memory, and progressive insanity. It usually appears in males in the fourth or fifth decade of life and is relentlessly progressive. Death occurs in 10–15 years after the first symptom appears. Individuals born into a family which suffers from Huntington's chorea should not reproduce since there is a very strong possibility that any offspring will also be affected. There is no treatment and the only way to deal with the condition is to allow the affected family to die out. Occasionally the condition occurs as a natural mutation in a family which has had no previous experience of the disease.

The affected person appears normal until middle life and it is difficult to believe that the degeneration will occur. However, the fact must be faced and the individual should be counselled regarding marriage and future progeny. Severe difficulties may arise when a marriage partner is unaware of the inherited nature of the disease. Any families which have an affected member must be made fully cognizant of the nature of the disease and must be helped to face the responsibilities that they have towards the community and society in which they live. Coping with an individual who has Huntington's chorea is not easy since the slow progressive nature of the condition indicates a long-term problem.

HYDROCEPHALUS

The brain and spinal cord are bathed in a fluid known as cerebrospinal fluid or C.S.F. This fluid is formed in channels, known as ventricles, within the brain substance. The C.S.F. flows through the channels and circulates around the brain and spinal cord continuously and in a constant amount regulated by absorption on the brain surface. If there is a block to circulation hydrocephalus results, the degree depending on the site and extent of the block. Cerebrospinal fluid accumulates in the ventricles and the increase in fluid volume, which may reach enormous proportions, causes the ventricles to dilate. Dilatation of the ventricles compresses the brain tissue surrounding them. In an infant and young child the skull bones are relatively soft and the internal pressure produced by the amount of fluid causes the head to enlarge. If hydrocephalus occurs in an older child the dilatation of ventricles and compression of brain tissues occur with no outward head enlargement.

Hydrocephalus may be due to congenital malformation and be present at birth. Postnatal infections such as meningitis can also cause narrowing and blockage of the communicating channels. Congenital hydrocephalus is usually associated with spina bifida. There may be an inheritance factor associated with congenital hydrocephalus. Symptoms include failure in development, spasticity, blindness, fits, and inability to lift the very large head. Sometimes the hydrocephalic process becomes arrested and intellectual development is normal. If the condition is progressive this causes mental deterioration due to severe brain damage. Hydrocephalus can be treated with reasonably good result. The main problem is the excess fluid, but if this can be drained the pressure on the brain is relieved. An artificial drain known as a Spitzhalter valve is inserted, which drains the C.S.F. into the blood-stream, so by-passing the normal channels and going directly into the venous system. A valve prevents backflow of blood into the brain. Drainage of fluid halts the process and, if done at an early stage, prevents the development of damage. There are complications regarding this method of treatment. The valve may become disconnected or blocked and infection may occur, entering at the site of insertion. Symptoms of complications include raised temperature, headaches, vomiting, and fits, and emergency treatment may be required.

Many children with hydrocephalus lead normal lives following treatment and cannot be distinguished from their peers. Some have other physical disabilities which are more trouble than the hydrocephalus. Some children with hydrocephalus have not received treatment early enough to prevent damage and may show marked retardation and other symptoms. Parents of children with this condition should be encouraged to allow them to lead a normal life and to avoid overprotection and undue anxiety. It is difficult to persuade parents to do this, but it is important to make sure that they understand the nature of the condition, the significance of symptoms should any arise, and the future prospects for the child. The problem of further children should also be discussed, if the parents wish it. If the hydrocephalus is congenital and particularly if associated with spina bifida there is a 1 in 12 chance that another child born to this family will suffer similar deformity.

HYPERTENSION

Hypertension or high blood-pressure occurs in many people, particularly in association with ageing. The pressure of blood as it flows through the body depends on two factors. The first is that the arteries are normally elastic and can expand to accommodate blood when it flows through. In later life many individuals have atherosclerotic changes (*see* ATHEROSCLEROSIS) in their blood-vessels and this reduces elasticity, causing a rise in measured blood-pressure. The other factor affecting blood-pressure is the pumping action of the heart and the volume of blood pumped out. A rise in blood-volume entering the arterial system increases blood-pressure. Increase in blood-volume occurs in thyrotoxicosis or in aortic valvular disease.

A certain degree of blood-pressure is essential to ensure an adequate blood-supply to all parts of the body. A raised blood-pressure may rupture blood-vessels which cannot cope with the increase in pressure. It may also cause heart failure, the heart being unable to continue pumping efficiently to overcome the resistance of the arteries. In most cases of hypertension there is no obvious cause although kidney disease and hormonal disturbances are likely to cause a rise in blood-pressure. Symptoms include headache, visual disturbances, dizziness, irritability, and palpitations.

Occasionally malignant hypertension occurs which proceeds rapidly to death. All symptoms are exaggerated. Blood-vessels in the eyes are often diseased and blindness may occur before death ensues.

Hypertension is a common cause of strokes (*see* CEREBRAL HAEMORRHAGE), particularly in old age. If the hypertension is diagnosed and treated this may prevent strokes occurring.

Treatment consists of drugs which have the ability to reduce the high levels to which blood-pressure may rise. Obesity is thought to aggravate hypertension and dieting is usually advised. Smoking causes constriction of blood-vessels and should be reduced or stopped. A busy working life associated with stress does not help to reduce blood-pressure and there should be a moderation in all activities with more rest and less worry.

There is an inherited tendency to develop hypertension. It appears to occur in several members of a family. Women appear to tolerate raised blood-pressure more than men, in whom it has more serious results. People with hypertension can be irritable and bad-tempered and often are responsible for family conflict and marital disharmony. The marriage partner should be made aware of the fact that these are symptoms of the condition so that allowances can be made. Marital squabbles only serve to cause a further rise in blood-pressure levels and further deterioration in health.

HYPOTHERMIA

All the processes that go on within the body require a certain temperature for normal activity. Normal body temperature is 37° C. (98·4° F.) and below 35° C. (95° F.) all physiological activity becomes impaired. Every activity slows down. At 28° C. (82·5° F.) life is no longer possible and death occurs.

Hypothermia occurs when heat loss exceeds heat production. In normal conditions if the temperature of the atmosphere drops the blood-vessels in the skin contract to conserve heat, more clothes are put on, hot food and drink are indulged in, and the temperature of the atmosphere is raised through some type of artificial heating such as an electric, gas, paraffin, or coal fire. However, there are certain circumstances when these precautions cannot be carried out and, because the body is not protected against heat loss, it loses excessive heat and the condition may become irreversible.

Hypothermia is particularly common in infants and in elderly infirm people. It occasionally occurs in others due to unforeseen mishaps. People living on their own who may go into diabetic coma, or who have an accident which leaves them unconscious, or who are in a disturbed condition due to the effect of drugs or alcohol may also suffer from the effects of cold and may be unable to take necessary preventive steps. Infants left out in cold weather or who sleep in unheated rooms are prone to hypothermia. Red cheeks may be deceptive and should be suspect unless proved otherwise. The temperature-regulation mechanism in babies takes time to mature and they should never be exposed to cold for long periods. The elderly person living alone on a small pension will often economize on fuel and food, and if infirm will tend not to move around too frequently. The cold may effect such a person insidiously and he or she may be unaware of mental and physical changes taking place until it is too late. Cold causes mental confusion which gradually lapses into coma.

Treatment of hypothermia may reverse the effects, but it may be irreversible by the time the person is discovered. The body should be warmed slowly by wrapping it in a blanket in a warm room. In the elderly, pneumonia is a complication and antibiotics should be given to prevent this. The person should also be examined for underlying illness causing the infirmity, e.g., diabetes, hypothyroidism.

This is a serious condition which is completely avoidable. However, many old people live on their own with very few visitors. Many have only a very limited amount of money to live on and economize on heat and food. Some have lost interest in life and no longer want to look after themselves. Some develop illnesses and are too weak to fetch a doctor; others become ill suddenly and have no time to fetch a doctor before they are unconscious. The plight of the lonely, elderly infirm is a very serious one. Increasing longevity raises the problem of loneliness. The community has a great responsibility in providing practical services for the elderly. Friendly visiting is important, as is the provision of accurate information about supplementary benefits that old people are entitled to. Warden services on housing estates provide a useful service, as do the residential homes for the elderly. Local authorities should be encouraged to use voluntary organizations in their efforts to give all old people comprehensive help and to make sure that they all benefit by available services.

ICHTHYOSIS

This condition is also known as fish-skin disease owing to the fact that the skin is scaly, dry, and hard. It is a congenital condition, but the symptoms may not appear until some months after birth. It is inherited and is found in several generations.

There is a layer on the skin surface called the horny layer which is continually being rubbed off and replaced. This layer makes the skin waterproof and prevents the entrance of bacteria into the body. Ichthyosis is due to abnormality of this horny layer. Vitamin A has some part to play in normal skin development and ichthyosis may also be due to some abnormality in vitamin-A metabolism. The basic defect is reduction of skin capacity for holding water and hence the intense dryness.

Symptoms include dry scaly hair and thickened nails. The whole body is covered in dirty grey scales. Complications include eczema. Treatment is by application of external creams, hot baths, and sun-bathing.

Ichthyosis sometimes develops in association with leprosy or malignant disease, particularly Hodgkin's disease.

The unsightliness of this skin condition gives rise to many problems. Avoidance by other people leads to social isolation which, in turn, leads to psychological trauma and emotional conflict. People with ichthyosis find difficulty in leading a normal life and find winter a particularly difficult time as it encourages further changing of the skin. Social workers must be prepared for a great deal of resistance to help since the condition is intractable and the person knows this. It is up to the professional worker to help the individual to come to terms with this disability which is a far greater handicap than many other more severe medical conditions. Any physical disability which is as obvious as a skin disease is liable to provoke a far greater aversion response in other people than severe disease hidden within the body or by heavy clothing. It will probably be difficult for any professional worker to cope with the unsightliness in the first instance as the condition makes the person look dirty and this is an added aversion factor.

ILEAL LOOP

The manufacture of an ileal loop is an operation which is performed to help overcome bladder problems seen particularly in relation to children with spina bifida. In this operation a loop of small intestine is separated from the rest of the intestine but not from its blood-supply. It is then brought to the external abdominal wall to form a spout. The ureters (channels leading from the kidney to the bladder) are separated from the bladder and transplanted into this loop so that urine passes through the spout in the abdominal wall. This operation alleviates persistent infection spreading from the paralysed bladder to the kidneys which can, in time, cause irreparable damage.

Appliances can be fitted over the spout and attached to the abdominal wall which will collect the urine and which can be emptied at intervals. The correct fitting of these appliances is necessary since it is important to ensure that the child remains clean and dry, both for medical and aesthetic reasons. Persistent skin wetness leads to soreness, ulceration, and infection leading to further misery for the child. Persistent urine leakage also leads to unpleasant smell and isolation of the child from his peers.

The problems of incontinence are once again highlighted. This is a particularly embarrassing problem for young people, especially at the time of adolescence, when every body function, however normal, becomes a source of embarrassment. Young people trying to establish themselves in an adult world, who have complications such as ileal loop and appliances, must be well trained in using them and learning how to live with them. The acceptance of this encumbrance is often far more difficult than the other complications of spina bifida. A teenager with this appliance will find it most difficult to make any type of sexual relationship unless it is with another spina bifida sufferer. As has been said elsewhere, children with spina bifida are normal young people with normal desires and feelings. They are going to face enormous frustration by not being able to fulfil these normal desires. An ileal loop and bag can complicate matters even further if the person who has these is unable to adjust to them.

INCONTINENCE OF URINE

Urine is produced in the kidneys and passed from these organs through two channels (the ureters) to the bladder. From the bladder urine reaches the exterior via the urethra.

The bladder is a muscular organ which is capable of being distended by an increasing volume of urine until the individual is suddenly aware of a feeling of wishing to void urine (micturition). Micturition can be postponed voluntarily by contraction of the muscle band found at the junction of the bladder and the urethra, known as the bladder sphincter. Control of micturition is an important developmental step in the process of natural maturation. It depends on an intact nervous system, and congenital malformation may prevent micturition control with consequent permanent incontinence. Control of micturition may also be lost, or become faulty, in later life due to damage or disease of the bladder and urethral musculature and surrounding organs, or to disease or damage of the nervous system. There is a spinal cord centre for the control of micturition and there is also a higher control centre in the brain. Damage or disease of the spinal cord below the micturition control centre leaves the micturition process undisturbed. Conditions causing partial or complete incontinence include local damage due to childbirth, prostatectomy, other pelvic operative procedures, or pelvic injury. Old age itself leads to degeneration of musculature and bladder muscle may become less efficient.

Spinal cord damage due to accident or injury usually leads to incontinence. Most paraplegics have the added problem of lack of micturition control although some learn methods whereby they can prevent constant trickling of urine. Nervous system diseases causing incontinence include multiple sclerosis, syphilis, and tumour of the spinal cord. Degeneration of the brain due to atherosclerosis may affect control centres and lead to incontinence. A common congenital malformation causing incontinence is spina bifida.

Urinary incontinence is one of the most difficult and distressing complications of any of the diseases or injuries mentioned above. A constant trickle of urine is an embarrassment and requires the wearing of waterproof garments at least. Most men wear some type of appliance to contain the urine. Sometimes a catheter is put permanently in position; other men wear external attachments which fit around the penis. The appliances for women are not so effective owing to the different anatomical disposition of the urinary apparatus. Where appliances are worn urine is collected in a bag which is emptied at intervals. Wearing the appliances may prove an embarrassment, particularly in children. In adults they can be concealed under clothing. If retention of urine is present as well as incontinence there is the added danger of back-pressure and damage to kidneys; and infection is a constant danger, particularly if a catheter is used. Bacteria are easily introduced and thrive in urine which lies stagnant in the bladder. Infection may pass to the kidneys and cause further damage. Despite appliances and waterproofing, people with incontinence are often wet and, if paralysis is also present, there is the ever-present danger of the development of pressure-sores (*see* BED-SORES). Another problem with incontinence is the difficulty with smell and cleanliness. Women in particular worry about this aspect and it can be a very real problem. Some people with incontinence live in houses without bathrooms or in accommodation where the bathroom is inaccessible. For these, many difficulties can be solved by seeing that a person suffering from incontinence is moved to the right sort of house with easy access to toilet and bathroom.

INFLUENZA

Influenza is a common, acute, and infectious illness caused by a group of viruses. It is characterized by the development of a high temperature, prostration, and a tendency to complications particularly in the lungs. Influenza occurs in epidemics at 4–5-year intervals, and it can also occur in sporadic cases.

The group of viruses which are responsible for influenzal illnesses are all related to each other but may cause symptoms to vary in individuals, depending upon which particular virus member of the group is responsible. The common symptoms that arise are headache, pains in limbs, loss of appetite, and shivering. Some individuals may develop vomiting and diarrhoea, others may exhibit symptoms referable to the respiratory tract, i.e., coughing and sneezing. The acute symptoms of influenza may last from 2 to 5 days after which there is usually complete recovery. However, there are certain factors which should be taken into consideration which make influenza an illness that should be treated with respect and not taken too lightly. The initial virus attack on the tissues makes them vulnerable to secondary invasion by foreign bacteria. These bacteria are able to enter the body at this time because of the weakened body defences consequent upon viral invasion. The lungs are particularly liable to secondary infection and acute bronchopneumonia may follow the initial influenzal illness. There are certain groups of people who are more likely to be at risk. These are the very old and the very young, and those suffering from chronic bronchitis, emphysema, bronchiectasis, and other chronic lung diseases where lung tissue is already damaged and where there is less reserve healthy tissue available. Also at risk are those with chronic heart conditions. Apart from the acute severe lung complications, meningitis, sinusitis, and middle-ear infections can all occur following influenza. The outcome of these complications can themselves lead to chronic illness and even to fatal results in those already weakened by previous long-term disease. Another serious side-effect of influenza is the condition known as post-influenzal depression which may occur during the convalescence period. This can be severe enough to cause suicide. In less dramatic cases this depression prolongs recovery and prevents return to work.

Vaccines are available which are not completely effective, are expensive to prepare, and are only useful for short-term protection. However, they are available to be used to prevent influenza in the vulnerable groups mentioned above. They are also used extensively in industry to prevent loss of time away from work.

INSULIN

Insulin is a hormone produced by the pancreas. The body is unable to utilize sugar without the presence of insulin and lack of this hormone is incompatible with life. Insulin causes removal of sugar from the blood-stream following the ingestion of food. It also helps in tissue formation and the storage of carbohydrate by the liver. High sugar-levels in blood stimulate the pancreas to produce insulin, which in turn reduces sugar-levels to normal.

Failure of insulin production leads to the development of diabetes mellitus (*see* DIABETES MELLITUS) and all the attendant complications of this deficiency disease. Lack of natural insulin may be due to disease of the pancreas. It may also be due to the fact that natural resources cannot keep pace with the large amounts of sugar ingested by the individual. Obese middle-aged and elderly ladies tend to develop a milder type of diabetes, which diet and weight reduction can cure. In these cases insulin is still available for normal requirements but not for the very excessive demands made by a gluttonous sweet tooth. Artificial insulins are available for those individuals who are no longer able to produce their own. The amounts required depend on the individual and his or her daily activities and diet.

Soluble insulin is a short-acting insulin which is often used in the initial stages of treatment when it is necessary to investigate individual requirements. Several injections are required daily. Children require soluble insulin since growing processes and bursts of activity make it difficult to estimate day-to-day requirements.

Protamine zinc insulin and zinc insulin suspensions are both designed for slow absorption over a longer period. These require only one injection daily. Sometimes soluble insulin is given with protamine zinc insulin to achieve a finer balance. Insulin zinc suspension consists of particles of different sizes, and by varying particle size the rate of absorption of insulin into the blood-stream can be controlled.

Artificial balance with insulin is a very delicate process. At the present time it is considered that insulin should be given in association with a strictly controlled sugar-free diet containing weighed amounts of carbohydrate, protein, and fats. Urine tests for sugar are carried out daily or weekly by the diabetics themselves and a raised sugar content usually indicates aberration of diet. Infections and illness can also cause abnormalities in urine-sugar content. Diabetic persons usually learn to adjust their own insulin intake and diet.

Side-effects of insulin therapy include overdose leading to coma, convulsions, and occasionally death. The brain needs sugar and if all sugar is removed from the blood-stream the brain ceases to function. Other side-effects include development of tumours or scarring at the site of injection (usually the thigh).

Treatment of the results of excess intake of insulin (hypoglycaemia) includes prevention—by making sure that meals are never missed and that the patient recognizes the early symptoms. Glucose should always be readily available for oral administration. If the person is unconscious when seen he will need immediate glucose injections into a vein. Recurrent hypoglycaemic attacks may lead to permanent brain damage with personality changes. This may happen if diabetes occurs in childhood. Hypoglycaemic attacks are very common during the juvenile and adolescent periods. They cease to be so important when growth ceases and the body matures.

IRON

This element is an essential component of the oxygen-transport system in the body. Haemoglobin, the pigment in red blood-cells, is comprised of iron linked with protein and is responsible for carrying oxygen to the tissues and for removing carbon dioxide from them.

Iron is normally obtained from the diet. It is released from food in the stomach and intestine and is absorbed into the body. Iron intake is controlled by the blood haemoglobin level and only the amount required to replace that lost by the body is absorbed. The rest is eliminated in the faeces. Foods rich in iron include liver, meat, and eggs.

Iron deficiency is usually due to abnormal bleeding and is common in women, particularly those who lose heavily during menstruation, and those who have abnormal bleeding episodes during pregnancy and childbirth. Iron deficiency also occurs after surgery, accident, or injury. Elderly people living alone and taking inadequate nutrition often develop iron deficiency or anaemia. Iron can be replaced by a diet rich in foods containing this element and by drug treatment. Iron tablets should be accompanied by vitamin C and protein as these encourage absorption of iron from the intestine. Occasionally iron by mouth is effective and iron is given by injection. Side-effects of iron injections include skin-staining and local tumours. Iron by mouth may give rise to diarrhoea and should be kept from young children as excess intake may cause death in infancy.

Excess iron in the body is usually due to failure of the normal blocking mechanism in the intestine and, therefore, to excess absorption. Absorption is normally controlled by haemoglobin levels and only a small amount passes through the intestine. When this mechanism fails up to ten times the usual amount may be absorbed and be deposited in body tissues in the form of the pigment haemosiderin. Failure in the absorption mechanism gives rise to the disease known as haemochromatosis, which is a chronic disease extending over many years. The main symptoms are due to destruction of various organs by deposition of haemosiderin. Diabetes is a common complication due to destruction of the pancreas. Heart damage also occurs and the liver and testicles are usually involved. The skin is heavily pigmented and the patient appears unusually bronzed. This condition tends to occur in men and there is a familial incidence. Women may develop the condition after the menopause. Excess iron can be removed by regular bleeding and complications such as diabetes are treated in the appropriate manner. The condition is not incompatible with normal working life unless the complications cause severe disability.

JAUNDICE

This is a symptom of disease. It is caused by the presence of excess amounts of the pigment bilirubin in the blood-stream. Bilirubin is a product of the breakdown of old red blood-cells and is normally contained in small amounts in the blood-stream. The rest is excreted, via the liver and bile-ducts, into the gastro-intestinal system and incorporated into the faeces.

Excess pigment may enter the blood-stream as a result of excess production or from blockage to the exit from the liver or the bile-ducts so that, instead of entering the intestine, it regurgitates into the blood-stream. If blood-cells are being abnormally destroyed more bilirubin may be produced than can be dealt with. This may occur in incompatible blood transfusions and abnormal blood conditions such as in sickle-cell anaemia, when the red blood-cells are an abnormal shape and are destroyed more easily. Drugs may cause abnormal destruction of red blood-cells and infections may also cause destruction of red blood-cells, e.g., malaria.

Normal amounts of pigment may be prevented from being removed to the intestines by blockage in the liver or in the bile-ducts. Severe liver damage causes jaundice.

Obstruction in the bile-ducts by stones, inflammation, or tumours may also cause jaundice.

Jaundice may be associated with other signs of liver damage including a tendency to haemorrhage, oedema, coma, and death. In gall-bladder disease jaundice is associated with very pale faeces, severe pain, and vomiting. Itching may accompany jaundice and in liver disease may be a very distressing symptom.

Jaundice occurs in babies. It may be a physiological accompaniment of birth and is then of no significance. Occasionally it is severe and is due to an incompatible blood reaction accompanied by abnormal breakdown of blood-cells. If the mother has Rhesus-negative blood and the baby is Rhesus positive (from the father) the two factors interact to cause red-cell destruction in the baby. The pigment is deposited in the tissues and, if it is deposited in the brain, can cause mental retardation and abnormalities of movement (*see* CEREBRAL PALSY). This can be avoided by immediate blood transfusion following birth.

THE KIDNEY

The kidney is the organ mainly responsible for removal of waste products from the body. Its function is the maintenance of normal blood composition, and excretion of abnormal substances will continue until blood composition returns to normal. Each individual possesses two kidneys.

The kidney acts as a filter and is not capable of chemically altering any substance which enters it. Blood passes through the organ and abnormal products of metabolism are filtered into the urine. The kidney also maintains normal water and salt balance. Excess water is normally filtered into the urine. If water and salts are lost by other means, e.g., by sweating through the skin, then the kidney will reduce the amount of water and salt in the urine to compensate for this.

The urine is the product of kidney filtration and is composed of water and waste products. It is usually a clear yellow fluid, the colour depending on the amount of water and the presence of pigments. In jaundice the colour of urine is altered by the presence of excess bile-pigments. Other diseases are responsible for the presence of abnormal substances in the blood and urine, and a simple urine test may indicate the presence of disease, e.g., sugar in diabetes.

Kidney failure leads to the accumulation of waste products in the blood-stream. The presence of these substances in increasing concentrations in the blood and body tissues is incompatible with life. The artificial kidney has been developed to filter the blood and remove waste products (*see* RENAL DIALYSIS).

LEPROSY

Leprosy is an infectious disease caused by a bacterium. It is not easily communicable and is only passed from one person to another by close contact over a long period. It is a very slowly progressive condition and is not usually responsible for death of affected individuals. It is characterized by skin destruction and it also attacks the nerves, causing loss of sensation, muscle weakness, and paralysis.

The leprosy bacterium is related to that causing tuberculosis. In both diseases the infant is very susceptible and should be removed from an infected parent at birth. The time between the bacterium entering the body and the exhibition of symptoms may be from 1 to several years.

There are two main types of leprosy known as tuberculous and lepromatous. In tuberculous leprosy symptoms are mostly referable to nerve damage and include loss of sensation, deformities, loss of fingers and toes, and gangrene. Lepromatous leprosy shows symptoms referable to skin damage and includes development of nodules, loss of eyebrows, and ulceration of the nose. There may also be patches of depigmentation of the skin and the individual affected has an appearance somewhat reminiscent of a lion.

Treatment is prolonged, but the condition can be cured by drug therapy in association with a good diet. Surgical treatment may be necessary to cope with gangrene and other deformities.

Leprosy is a difficult disease to treat in this country. It is on the increase owing to immigration from those countries where the condition is common. In many cases the person feels reasonably well and it is difficult to keep him isolated and out of employment. For some people leprosy has strong connotations with lack of cleanliness and sinfulness, particularly for those who have deep religious feelings. It is often difficult for such people to come to terms with their disease and they may go through periods of deep depression, self-recrimination, and suicidal tendencies. When the disease is diagnosed it is important for the condition to be carefully explained and to try to make the individual understand the nature of his disease. Biblical associations make it a hard task, particularly where the individual is semiliterate and from a culture different to that of his adopted country. The problem is complicated by the length of time required for cure and the fact that medication must be adhered to without constant hospital surveillance. Regular follow-up visits are needed to give the patient support and to make sure drugs are being taken.

LEUKAEMIA

White blood-cells are responsible for body defences against bacterial invasion and attack by other substances toxic to the body. Without these cells the body soon succumbs to overwhelming infection. Tissues producing these cells include bone-marrow, lymph-glands, and spleen. Occasionally an abnormal change occurs in these tissues and normal tissue is replaced by malignant or cancerous cells which multiply rapidly and cause a failure in production of normal white cells.

Although the basic cause for this change is unknown it is thought that X-rays and other nuclear radiation may increase the susceptibility of the individual to the development of cancer of those tissues concerned with the formation of white blood-cells. This is a type of cancer and is known as leukaemia. Some leukaemias are thought to be due to viruses. It is not thought that there is any inherited tendency for development of this condition.

Leukaemia may be acute or chronic. Acute leukaemia occurs mainly in children and young adults and usually has a rapid course to fatality. Death may be postponed by the use of drugs and blood transfusion, but there is, on the whole, a poor response to treatment. Symptoms include general debility and loss of weight, spontaneous haemorrhages, and anaemia. A severe acute infection which is unresponsive to treatment may be the first indication of the presence of leukaemia.

Chronic leukaemia is a disease of older people and, as the name suggests, has a more prolonged course over several years before death ensues. Symptoms are similar to those of acute leukaemia with enlargement of liver, spleen, and other lymph-glands. Treatment is by drug therapy, radiotherapy, and blood transfusion. Occasionally cortisone is found to be useful in treatment.

At the present time death is an inevitable accompaniment of leukaemia and is particularly rapid in acute leukaemia. Parents of children with this condition find it very hard to accept that their child, previously so healthy, is now doomed. They require a great deal of support from the social worker and are often not willing to accept this help. It is natural that they should refuse to accept the idea of death as far as their child is concerned and remission due to treatment often leads them into false hopes. Naturally, each case must be considered individually, but it is important that from the outset no false hopes are raised and that the parents understand the probable outcome. People in the same predicament often gain comfort from each other and it is a useful exercise to encourage groups of parents to meet and discuss their fears and difficulties.

Older people with leukaemia also have their problems. They now must face the possibility of death and this should not be avoided. People who are facing death often want to discuss it with someone and this opportunity should not be denied them. The doctor or professional social worker cannot cope with this problem until he has come to terms with death himself. Many people assume that the subject of death should never be mentioned but should be avoided at all costs. This is a fallacy: death is a subject that should be broached openly but with sensitivity. There will be remissions with chronic leukaemia as with the acute form. The person should be encouraged to lead a normal life during these periods and to enjoy himself to the best of his ability. Chronic disease gives both the patient and the relatives time to accept the inevitable. It is important to make sure that both the individual and the relatives understand the nature of the condition and the eventual outcome so that they can make the best use of the time available.

LUNGS

The lungs serve as organs of air exchange, allowing oxygen to enter and carbon dioxide to leave the blood-stream. There are two lungs, consisting of tissue composed of alveoli, i.e., large hollow cells with thin walls in close contact with blood-capillaries. Clusters of alveoli are connected to bronchioles and bronchi which lead from the mouth, nose, and trachea to the lung tissue and vice versa. The lungs are passive organs which cannot contract and dilate independently. They expand owing to movement of the chest wall and diaphragm. When the chest wall moves out and the diaphragm moves down this increases the negative pressure in the chest cavity and the lungs expand, drawing air in. When the chest wall and diaphragm return to their resting positions the lungs deflate and air is expired. The lungs are surrounded by a lubricated membrane which is continuous with that lining the chest wall. It is known as the pleura.

The lungs have a profuse blood-supply, the pulmonary circulation, which is responsible for the adequate gaseous exchange necessary for the efficient functioning of all body tissues. Deoxygenated blood flows through the lungs in close proximity to the alveoli or air sacs and receives an oxygen supply. Oxygenated blood then returns from the lungs to the left side of the heart via the pulmonary veins.

In order that this system should function adequately the alveolar walls and capillary walls must be intact. In disease processes attacking the alveolar walls these are thickened, broken down, and made irreparable which reduces the respiratory surface, i.e., that area available for air exchange. This may cause respiratory embarrassment to a minor or major degree. When the lungs are severely disabled this affects the heart and circulatory system. A damaged lung prevents free flow of blood and this causes pressure on the right side of the heart with consequent right-sided heart failure.

MULTIPLE SCLEROSIS

Multiple sclerosis is a disease of the central nervous system. Nervous tissue is covered in a fatty sheath composed of a substance known as myelin. In multiple sclerosis the myelin sheath undergoes degeneration in patches and this causes interruption in the transmission of nerve impulses. These patches of demyelination can occur in any part of the nervous system and, consequently, symptoms of the disease show a great deal of variation from one individual to another. However, the initial symptoms are usually similar. Unexplained transient blurring of vision or double vision, with or without eye pain, may herald development of the disease although it may be some years before further symptoms appear. Weakness and loss of sensation in limbs may be the first sign of the disease. The condition is also characterized by remissions and relapses, recovery of function appearing to take place and remissions lasting for long periods of up to 20 years. In some cases there may be no remission, but a gradual deterioration with increasing disability. In others, premature death may occur due to infection. In children, a particularly malignant form of the disease may occur which proves rapidly fatal. The commonest age of onset is in the range from 20 to 50 years and women tend to be afflicted more than men.

The cause of the disease is obscure: viruses, heredity, climate, and diet have all been cited as factors by various researchers. As yet no definite agent has been discovered.

As the disease progresses the person becomes more disabled with weakness and paralysis of the lower limbs necessitating a wheel-chair life, loss of control of bladder and bowels, blindness, mental deterioration, and speech difficulties. Many patients with severe disability exhibit a euphoric state showing little concern for their condition. This is thought to be a compensating mechanism. Others are not so cheerful and suicide attempts may occur. Some develop psychiatric complications.

Rehabilitation should be attempted during remission, including attendance at Handicapped Persons' Centres, participation in social activities and, if possible, return to employment. It is important to avoid the development of bed-sores and urinary infections which are common accompaniments of incontinence. As far as pregnancy is concerned, multiple sclerosis seems to worsen after childbirth. But termination and sterilization may cause added stress and exacerbation of the illness so it is probably best to allow pregnancy to continue. If possible a woman with multiple sclerosis should avoid conception.

Good health and working capacity may be maintained for many years if the relapses are not too severe. Stress should always be avoided and rest is very important. No one with multiple sclerosis should be allowed to tire unduly.

This is a difficult disease to cope with owing to the uncertainty of its development. Relatives should be aware of the worst that can happen but should not treat the person who has multiple sclerosis as a disabled imbecile. A normal life should be attempted within the limits of the capacities of the individual. Obviously this will be very limited in many cases. The disease is a long-drawn-out one with many complications and setbacks. It takes great fortitude to cope with a person suffering from multiple sclerosis, and relatives, as well as the individual affected, need a great deal of help.

MUSCULAR DYSTROPHY

Muscular dystrophy is a muscle-wasting disease which occurs mainly in boys and which is inherited. There are several different types, some less severe than others. Sensation in the muscles remains the same and it is only movement that is affected. It is the female who carries the abnormal characteristic. She passes it on to half the sons that she has, i.e., there is a 50–50 chance that a son born to an affected mother will suffer from muscular dystrophy. There is also a 50–50 chance that a daughter of such a mother will be a carrier for the disease. It is very rare that a girl develops the disease and, if so, it is by a different pathway of inheritance.

The child appears to develop normally until the age of 3 or 4. There is then progressive difficulty in walking and sitting, and the child falls often. Muscles of the thighs and legs appear to be enlarged, but in reality they are infiltrated with fatty tissue and are weak. Walking is progressively difficult and finally the child becomes confined to a wheel-chair. The facial muscles are affected and the hands may be weak. Death occurs prematurely due to failure of respiratory muscles or chest infection. Degrees of severity are seen in this condition and some boys survive into the second and third decade, becoming progressively disabled until they are completely dependent.

The brain is not affected in this condition and the whole range of intellect can be seen in those suffering with muscular dystrophy. It is important to develop as many intellectual activities as possible for such young people since they will have to rely more and more on brain activity as their bodies fail them. Some people with muscular dystrophy have attended colleges and universities and have worked for a period. Obviously employment will be limited. Parents with such children must be aware of the prognosis, but should be encouraged to give their child as normal a life as possible. Further pregnancies should be avoided if possible unless parents are prepared to take a 50–50 chance on having a further afflicted child. The fact that a young person with muscular dystrophy has a normal intellect makes it more difficult in many cases for acceptance and adjustment to the disability, particularly as they feel themselves deteriorating. They may need a great deal of support, particularly as they reach adolescence and begin to develop normal male feelings regarding the opposite sex, future employment, and careers.

MYASTHENIA GRAVIS

Myasthenia gravis is a disease in which the main symptom is excessive muscle weakness. Normally, stimulation of a nerve causes the release of a substance known as acetylcholine at the nerve ending which in time causes contraction of the particular muscle-fibre stimulated. The normal process is for the acetylcholine produced to cause muscle contraction and then to be destroyed by the action of an antagonistic substance. In myasthenia gravis it is thought that there is excess production of the antagonist and the acetylcholine is destroyed too rapidly. This causes undue muscle fatigue. Inheritance factors are not certain, although occasionally the disease appears in several members of a family.

Symptoms include double vision, difficulties with chewing and swallowing, and weakness of limb muscles. The most serious complication is failure of respiratory muscles with death from asphyxia resulting. There may be natural remisssions and a 20-year survival rate is not uncommon. Treatment is by administration of prostigmine, a substance which antagonizes the substance that causes the breakdown of acetylcholine.

It is thought that the thymus gland may have some role to play in this condition but it is not certain how. The condition is also sometimes associated with hyperthyroidism. It is certainly more common in women.

This is a very distressing condition which can be disabling. The discovery of adequate therapy has improved the outlook for survival, but the disease still puts limitations on the way of life for anyone suffering with myasthenia gravis. If the question of marriage and a family does arise, it can only be said that inheritance factors have not been proved. But the strain of bringing up a child or children is an added risk to the adequate control of the condition.

MYXOEDEMA

Partial or complete loss of thyroid activity leads to the development of myxoedema, a condition that is the complete opposite to hyperthyroidism (*see* THYROTOXICOSIS) although persistent overactivity of the thyroid can finally exhaust the gland and give rise to myxoedema. If a child is born with no thyroid gland and if this is not diagnosed, mental defects and stunted growth occur giving rise to a 'cretin'.

The disease is seen mainly in women who are reaching the menopause and symptoms are due to a general slowing down of all metabolic processes in the body. These include abnormal sensitivity to cold, loss of hair, slowness of movement, poor appetite and constipation, anaemia, menstrual problems, and slowed brain activity including the development of psychiatric conditions. The symptoms may be present in varying degrees depending on the amount of thyroid left functioning.

The condition, once recognized, can be treated adequately by replacement therapy. Thyroid hormone must be taken regularly and permanently in adequate dosage to restore normal body functions. Overdose of thyroid hormone leads to all the signs of thyrotoxicosis including palpitation, angina, and cardiac failure.

Sometimes the diagnosis of myxoedema can be overlooked, particularly if this develops over a prolonged period. An elderly person may become slow and confused and this may be taken as the natural degeneration expected in old age. However, anyone who appears with some or all of the symptoms attributable to thyroid deficiency should have specific investigations in order to exclude the possibility. In general it is not necessary for every ageing person to become demented, confused, and physically slow just because of age. Old age can be as healthy a period as infancy. All signs and symptoms of disease should be as thoroughly investigated in the elderly as in any other age-group. It is as important for this group of people to be as healthy as possible, particularly as many of them live alone and need all the faculties that they have to be in the best possible condition. Relatives may not notice the deterioration of an individual if they see him or her frequently and this is why myxoedema may be missed for a long time. Regular health checks and screening clinics can avoid this and—although there is some difference of opinion regarding the value of these screening services, particularly from the point of view of finding diseases in people who feel perfectly healthy—it certainly avoids a great deal of future misery if diseases and defects can be treated at an early stage in development.

NEPHRITIS

Nephritis, or inflammation of the kidneys, may occur in acute or chronic form. Inflammation is usually due to infection by the bacteria known as streptococci. The bacteria attack the throat causing soreness and fever and this is followed 6–10 days later by kidney symptoms. The body produces substances called antibodies to combat the bacterial invasion of the throat and these antibodies are deposited in the kidneys, giving rise to acute nephritis. The disease is common in young people, although it is seen in all age-groups.

The kidney is responsible for regulation of water and salt content in the body. In acute nephritis the kidney is no longer able to fulfil its functions properly and many of the symptoms are due to the retention of water and salt in the body. These symptoms include a raised blood-pressure and oedema (*see* OEDEMA). Other symptoms include blood in the urine (haematuria), headache, and back pain. Retention of large quantities of fluids in the body gives rise to further serious complications including heart enlargement and failure, lung congestion (pulmonary oedema), and brain damage. Oedema of the lungs gives rise to respiratory distress and brain oedema causes fits and coma. The treatment of acute nephritis is non-specific but includes bed-rest and restriction of fluid, salt, and protein.

Sometimes the kidneys fail completely, and the patient is treated by means of an artificial kidney. Drugs are also used to reduce blood-pressure, relieve heart failure, and remove excess fluid from the body. In most people recovery is complete and the kidneys return to normal function. However, in 15 per cent of cases complete recovery does not occur, and over the years there is gradual kidney destruction with the development of chronic nephritis and renal failure.

The majority of throat infections are not followed by the development of acute nephritis and it is not advisable to treat every sore throat with antibiotics. There are some people who are particularly susceptible to infection by the streptococcal bacteria and it is these who should receive special medical care and attention to avoid recurrence of kidney infection; second attacks are not uncommon in those who have previously suffered from acute nephritis.

OBESITY

Body-weight is controlled by various factors including the appetite centres situated in the brain, the activity of the thyroid and pituitary glands, and the activity of the glands associated with sexual function, i.e., ovaries and testicles. Even when all these control mechanisms are working normally, other factors have to be taken into consideration. These include occupation, greed, social circumstances, habit formation, and psychological disturbances. It is the second set of circumstances which are most important in the development of obesity since it is very rare that excess weight is caused by glandular imbalance or brain damage.

Some occupations are conducive to the development of obesity, for instance cooking and working in food factories or shops. It is very easy to develop a habit of eating between meals, or eating carbohydrate rather than protein and fatty foods. Some people eat when they are worried or upset and run to food as a comforter. Once obesity has developed it is difficult to overcome although not impossible.

There are three main types of food in the diet: carbohydrates, fats, and protein. Carbohydrates include bread, cakes, sweets, puddings, and chocolate. Proteins include meat, fish, eggs, and cheese. Fats include butter and margarine. These must all be taken as part of a balanced diet. If too much carbohydrate is consumed obesity will result. In this country carbohydrate foods are consumed in great amounts, to the detriment of health.

Obesity is unsightly, but it can also give rise to serious health hazards including diabetes, osteo-arthritis, varicose veins, heart degeneration, and aggravation of chronic bronchitis. It can predispose to complications in acute infections, and the prognosis of the outcome of surgery in an obese person is not good.

Treatment is difficult since it relies on the individual to carry out instructions. The only permanent way to cure obesity is by permanent watching of diet and with many people it is difficult to change the habits of a lifetime. Sometimes appetite-reducing drugs may help but some are habit-forming and others are known to have unpleasant side-effects.

Exercise is of little use but may make the person feel that he is doing something positive. It gives encouragement to see weight-loss following dieting effort and, in some cases, the administration of a drug will cause loss of fluid and consequent weight-loss. However, this should not be continued for long since fluid lost in this way is quickly regained. Eating encourages appetite and abstention from eating eventually leads to loss of appetite. People who persevere with dieting all say that they no longer want to eat a great deal.

Obesity is particularly difficult when it occurs in a teenager. The psychological problems present at this time of life can be severely complicated by obesity and the misery engendered may lead to gaining comfort by eating, this setting up a vicious circle. Young people should never be encouraged to eat large quantities of food, particularly carbohydrate, and mothers who stand over their growing children and force food down them out of misguided good intentions may be doing untold harm to them.

Anyone who is 20 per cent overweight at the time of an insurance examination has a weighted premium to pay which rises as obesity increases, for life expectancy is shortened in obese people. Such persons need practical help to combat an abnormal condition that is harmful to health.

OEDEMA

Excess fluid or fluid collected in an abnormal situation in the body is referred to as oedema. Normally body fluids are in equilibrium so that normal concentrations of these are maintained. Fluid in the blood-vessels is under constant pressure to escape, but the protein content of this fluid has a tendency to draw fluid into the blood-vessels from the tissues and these two forces balance each other. Another factor to be taken into consideration is the permeability of the blood-vessel wall. Under some conditions the vessel wall becomes abnormally porous and allows fluid to leak out.

The pressure in the blood-capillaries is increased if blood-flow is slowed down. This occurs where varicose veins are present (*see* VARICOSE VEINS) or, more generally, if the heart is failing and not pumping efficiently blood will flow more slowly around the body and capillary pressure will increase, upsetting the equilibrium and allowing fluid to escape.

Plasma proteins exert a pressure, drawing fluid into the vessels. If plasma proteins are reduced the pressure is reduced and more fluid remains in the tissues. Plasma proteins are reduced in kidney disease when the kidneys cannot conserve protein and a great deal is lost in the urine.

Damage to the capillary walls allows them to become porous. This occurs in local injury and in allergic reactions, e.g., in nettle rash.

Symptoms associated with oedema include swelling in certain parts of the body. In cardiac failure oedema can be demonstrated in most areas. In varicose veins oedema is permanent in the ankles and legs. Pressure on the swollen area produces an indentation which remains present for some time. This is known as pitting. In severe cases of cardiac failure the lungs become oedematous, giving rise to respiratory distress.

Generalized oedema can be treated with drugs known as diuretics. These cause the kidneys to excrete large quantities of water and so relieve oedematous distress. They must be used in conjunction with potassium tablets since excess potassium may be lost in diuresis and this can affect heart action (*see* POTASSIUM).

Oedema may occur in pregnancy, often in association with high blood-pressure. Fingers and legs are particularly prone to this type of oedema and a tight wedding ring indicates the need for immediate investigation. The combination of oedema and high blood-pressure is known as toxaemia and can be a serious complication of pregnancy.

Oedema may occur in brain tissue, particularly after brain injury. It can also occur in the brain in cardiac failure. Excess fluid in brain tissues gives rise to confusion, drowsiness, delirium, and coma.

OSTEO-ARTHRITIS

This condition is due to degeneration in the joints. It is a common accompaniment of ageing, but is prone to occur in joints which have had previous damage due to infection, inflammation, or injury. There is an hereditary factor, osteo-arthritis often occurring in several members of the same family.

Symptoms are due to wear and tear within the joint and may lead to severe disability. Pain and swelling occur in the affected joint and there is severe limitation of movement. Weight-bearing joints are particularly affected since these are the ones most subject to damage, i.e., hip, shoulder, and ankles. Obesity aggravates the problem as do dampness, anxiety, and depression. Osteo-arthritis often improves if the afflicted individual can move to a dry, warm climate. It is important to encourage dieting and to avoid injury to the joints. Aspirin helps to combat pain and there are other drugs which can also be used although they must be administered with caution, e.g., phenylbutazone and indomethacin. People with osteo-arthritis are often in great pain and tend to take more tablets than they should. Although overdose of aspirin may occur they are the safest of all the drugs used by those affected with the condition.

Surgery is used extensively to promote mobility, but not all patients are suitable for artificial replacement of joints. Other treatment includes injection of cortisone into the joint to relieve inflammation and the removal of abnormal fluid from joint spaces. A new treatment is the injection of silicone fluids into the joints. It is thought that one of the main reasons for the development of disability due to osteo-arthritis is the loss of joint fluid.

Replacement by silicone oils appears to lubricate the joint and can be responsible for a remarkable recovery of joint function.

It is most important to maintain mobility. This can be aided by intensive physiotherapy including heat and exercise, infra-red heat, and other physiotherapy treatment. Splints, collars, and other appliances can also help to improve and maintain mobility. Aids and adaptations in the home, usually provided by the local authority, can serve to relieve strains and stresses of daily life and to allow for independent living.

Gradually increasing disability and reduced mobility give rise to a great deal of distress in those afflicted by the condition of osteo-arthritis. In many cases the person will be elderly and may have only elderly relatives or an elderly marriage partner to call on for support. This raises the whole problem of limitation of mobility and dependence on others and can give rise to much family conflict and also lead to psychiatric illness. It is important to diagnose the condition early so that severe disability may be avoided.

PARAPLEGIA

Weakness or complete loss of use of both limbs, often associated with bladder and bowel disturbance, is known as paraplegia. Disease or injury may cause this and it may occur suddenly or develop over a prolonged period of time. The basic cause is damage to the part of the spinal cord responsible for control of the lower limbs with destruction of nervous tissue. In most cases once nervous tissue is destroyed it cannot be regenerated and damage is permanent.

Acute paraplegia is usually due to injury or accident, although it can also occur with tumours or other diseases of the nervous system, e.g., multiple sclerosis. Gradual onset of paraplegia may be due to multiple sclerosis, atherosclerosis with reduction of blood-supply to nervous tissue, and spinal cord compression due to tumour or injury. Acute and chronic paraplegia show the same end-result with wasting of the legs, contraction of the muscles, and bladder incontinence. If the contracted muscles are not actively treated by physiotherapy the legs will become deformed and permanently set in distorted positions.

Other complications of paraplegia include bladder difficulties. The paralysed bladder becomes overdistended with persistent wetting of the patient. There is back-pressure on the kidneys with resultant damage to the kidney.

There is often infection of the urine, bladder, and kidneys due to the stagnation of urine. The patient may be taught to empty his bladder by abdominal pressure. In some cases it is possible to develop automatic emptying by training. Others need to wear an indwelling catheter or other appliance permanently to drain urine from the bladder to the exterior.

Antibiotic therapy is often needed to treat bladder infections.

Bed-sores are a problem and a patient with paraplegia must move frequently and be turned every 2 hours during the night. Bed-sores are encouraged to develop by urine continually leaking and wetting the skin and urine control thus improves the chances of avoiding bed-sores.

People with paraplegia have many problems. If associated with progressive disease it is complicated by other symptoms of the disease; if due to accident it is an entity in itself. Many people lead relatively normal lives from wheel-chairs. Some marry and have families. Many men are able to have erections and ejaculations and can fertilize their wives. Women with paraplegia are capable of having children although they usually need Caesarean section for delivery.

Rehabilitation is very important. In paraplegia due to accident the body above the waist is usually normal, and all types of professions and jobs are open to people in wheel-chairs provided they are prepared to train and obtain the necessary qualifications. Special aids and adaptations may make all the difference to a paraplegic and transform his life from disability to normality. Many paraplegics are expert athletes and can take part in all sorts of sports including archery, swimming, and hockey. In the early weeks and months after the development of paraplegia the individual may suffer reactive depression, be pessimistic, and give up hope. It is during this time that he or she will require support and encouragement and need to see how other people in similar positions manage. Relatives also require encouragement during the initial period and for some considerable time afterwards.

THE PITUITARY GLAND

This is a small gland situated within the skull cavity underlying the brain tissue and connected by nerve-fibres to that part of the brain known as the hypothalamus. It also underlies the optic nerves. The gland is divided into anterior and posterior lobes, and is responsible for the secretion of several hormones vital to normal body function. It is commonly known as the master gland since it is responsible for control of the other endocrine glands in the body. Secretion of these hormones is controlled by the hypothalmus in response to normal concentrations in the blood-stream.

The anterior lobe of the pituitary gland secretes hormones responsible for control of the thyroid hormones, the adrenal cortical hormones, and the ovarian and testicular hormones. Hormones are also produced controlling growth and lactation. The posterior lobe is responsible for secretion controlling the output of water from the body and for milk ejection during breast-feeding.

Various diseases affect the pituitary gland and alter hormone secretion. Tumours of the anterior lobe are found which may cause deficiency in production, or overproduction, of anterior lobe hormones; surrounding brain tumours may infiltrate into the pituitary; and pressure from a diseased, enlarging pituitary gland can affect the optic nerves and cause visual damage leading to blindness.

Gigantism and acromegaly are both diseases due to excessive production of growth hormone, most often caused by primary tumour of the anterior lobe. Gigantism occurs in children before the bones stop growing and there is abnormal growth to excessive heights. Weakness and lethargy may accompany this condition since the pituitary gland sometimes degenerates following its excessive activity.

Acromegaly is the same disease occurring in adulthood when the bones have ceased to grow. They become thickened and enlarged. The face shows enlargement of all features, particularly of the lower jaw. The hands and feet grow in size. Other organs also enlarge and death may be due to heart enlargement and failure. Treatment is difficult: in some cases there is natural arrest of the disease; in children radiotherapy may help; and in adults the present method of treatment is to implant radioactive substances within the pituitary to try to slow down pituitary activity.

Hypopituitarism is also known as Simmonds' disease. It is most common following severe haemorrhage after childbirth, but can also be caused by pituitary destruction due to tertiary syphilis or tuberculosis. Symptoms are due to failure of all endocrine glands because of lack of pituitary stimulation. They include lethargy and cold intolerance attributable to lack of thyroid hormone, genital atrophy and failure to re-establish menstruation due to lack of sex hormones, reduced blood-sugar, sodium depletion, and water retention due to lack of adrenal cortical hormone. A typical waxy or alabaster pallor is also present although anaemia is not a symptom. Treatment is by eradication of the primary cause, if possible, and replacement with artificial hormones.

Pituitary dwarfism may be due to a congenital deficiency of growth hormones or to a tumour which destroys the cells producing this hormone. This type of dwarfism is associated with lack of development of secondary sexual characteristics but is compatible with a normal life-span. Treatment with injections of growth hormone is in the experimental stage.

The posterior pituitary may be affected by secondary deposits of tumour or by pressure from surrounding tumour. This causes reduction in output of the hormone regulating water content in the body and symptoms include output of large quantities of dilute urine, intense thirst, and consumption of large quantities of fluid. This disturbs rest and daily life to an intolerable degree. Treatment consists of removal of the basic cause and, if necessary, replacement therapy with appropriate amounts of the hormone concerned.

Loss of the pituitary gland without replacement therapy is incompatible with life.

POLIOMYELITIS

Poliomyelitis is an acute infectious illness which may give rise to serious long-term effects in severe cases. The disease is caused by a group of related viruses, any one of which may be responsible for an attack. Although originally the condition was most common in infants, hence the term infantile paralysis, in more recent years it has become most common in the 6–12 years age-range. Adults may also be affected.

The virus is excreted in the faeces of infected persons and may be spread via flies or human hands to food, water, or milk. It can enter the body through the digestive tract or it can be inhaled and enter via the respiratory tract. In either case, entry of the virus into the body may give rise to infection. Initial symptoms are those of an influenzal-type illness, i.e., headache, high temperature, shivering, vomiting, and pains in the limbs. However, the virus has a special predilection for the anterior horns of the spinal column, i.e., those parts of the cord responsible for voluntary muscle control. The virus may also attack the brain-stem, particularly those areas responsible for the central control of respiratory and circulatory function, and give rise to the severest form of poliomyelitis, i.e., bulbar palsy.

The results of viral attack may take one of several forms. The attack may be so mild as to go unnoticed, i.e., sub-clinical attack. This confers immunity from further attack without causing any damage to body tissues. A more severe infection may give rise to the above-mentioned influenzal-type illness without any further untoward symptoms. This type of infection also confers immunity to further attack. The most severe form of the infection occurs when paralysis follows the initial symptoms. If the paralysis occurs in groups of muscles responsible for essential function, e.g., the respiratory muscles, the outcome may be fatal. In cases of bulbar palsy central control of respiration and circulation may fail and 80 per cent of these cases have a fatal outcome. People with respiratory paralysis may survive due to artificial respiratory methods, but may spend the rest of their lives in an iron lung. Paralysis often occurs in groups of muscles which have, prior to infection, been subjected to hard work, e.g., the legs of an athlete or the hands of a pianist. One or more limbs may be affected, and in some cases the person may be confined to a wheel-chair for the rest of his life. Once muscle power is lost it is rarely recoverable. Selective paralysis of groups of muscles give rise to imbalance of action and may result in deformity, particularly of the spine. During convalescence physiotherapy is important in order to prevent contracture and deformities and to strengthen weakened muscles.

The condition is non-progressive. Once the initial damage is done and the infection overcome the loss of muscle power remains static. In later life arthritis is more prone to occur in those limbs affected but this is part of the degenerative process of ageing and is not unique to poliomyelitis victims. Physiotherapy, exercise, and general care of paralysed limbs help to prevent any premature degenerative processes.

A vaccine has been developed which is extremely effective and which is eliminating poliomyelitis as a cause of chronic disability in this country. The vaccine is administered orally at the age of 6 months in three doses at monthly intervals. This is a very acceptable preventive procedure and has been added to the list of routine immunization procedures in infancy.

POTASSIUM

This element is essential if the body is to function normally. It is found mainly in body tissues and the most important source of external supply is via food intake. Most common foods contain a certain amount. Potassium is excreted in the urine and faeces. Increase in excretion occurs when body tissues are broken down, e.g., in malnutrition or injury. Increased potassium may also occur in disease. The adrenal cortex is responsible for the control of potassium balance and excess production of adrenal hormones, due to tumour or after disease, increases the amount of potassium excreted from the body. Failure of the kidney to retain potassium due to kidney disease is another cause of excess loss. When there is a deficiency of adrenal hormones, potassium will be retained in abnormally high quantities (*see* ADDISON'S DISEASE). Diarrhoea causes massive loss of potassium and this can cause death. It is particularly dangerous in infants.

Potassium is required for normal heart action and other muscle activities. Heart failure can be a result of both excess and deficient amounts of potassium in the body. Deficiency also causes general muscular weakness and incapacity.

Familial periodic paralysis is a rare disease which is inherited and symptoms are caused by recurrent low levels of potassium. In heart failure and kidney failure and also in injury potassium is found in excess of the normal concentration. Excess potassium in the blood-stream will cause cessation of heart action.

PSORIASIS

This is a skin disease which is most inclined to make its first appearance in adolescence. It can affect any part of the body in any degree of severity and a first attack is usually followed by recurrences at regular intervals throughout life. There is a strong inheritance factor with the disease, which often occurs in different generations and in more than one member of the same generation. Symptoms include red scaly patches, particularly prone to develop on the elbows and knees and also on the scalp. There is a form of psoriasis which is associated with a severe arthritis of the fingers and other joints, but this is not common.

Various factors may cause a recurrence, including emotional disturbance, shock, illness, or injury. Pregnancy and childbirth may also cause an increase in severity of symptoms although it sometimes works in the opposite direction and the skin lesions clear during this period. A raised temperature sometimes causes disappearance of symptoms.

Remedies are external and include various ointments containing tar. Steroid applications may help and ultraviolet light can alleviate.

The problems associated with psoriasis are those of emotional stress occasioned by an unsightly disease. People tend to avoid unsightliness and skin conditions are particularly prone to cause this avoidance reaction. This is a particular difficulty when the disease attacks young girls and women. Emotional crises can exacerbate symptoms and an increase in severity of symptoms excites emotional disturbance. Thus the whole matter becomes a vicious circle. Sedative drugs can help to dampen emotions regarding the disease and may cause a remission of symptoms. Psoriasis is a chronic recurring disease and anyone suffering with it has to learn to come to terms with the affliction.

As there is a strong hereditary factor the problem of prospective parenthood must be taken into account. To a certain extent the attitude of parents will depend on how much they have suffered themselves from the effects of the disease as to how they feel about the possible production of a child with the same condition.

PULMONARY EMBOLUS

An embolus is a blood-clot which has broken off from the parent clot and has travelled to other parts of the body, particularly to the lungs. The parent clot, or thrombus, is usually found in the veins of the leg or pelvic area. Thrombosis in these veins is encouraged by a slowed rate of flow which occurs during immobilization following surgery, injury, or other illness. Women often develop venous thromboses following childbirth when damage may occur in the pelvic and leg veins. Venous blood returning to the lungs for reoxygenation carries emboli from the legs or pelvis and these tend to lodge in the blood-vessels of the lung.

Pulmonary emboli may be large and block a main vessel causing almost immediate death unless rapid emergency action is taken. Blockage of smaller vessels may not be fatal but may presage further episodes and are a warning for action to be taken. Symptoms include severe chest pain and breathlessness with feelings of anxiety and impending death. Sometimes there is blood-stained sputum. The severity of symptoms depends on the relative importance of the particular artery blocked by the embolus. If a large artery is blocked, it is imperative that the clot be removed immediately by surgery and that anticoagulant drugs be given, also immediately, to prevent further emboli developing.

Prolonged immobilization in bed for whatever reason is an added hazard to life and should be avoided. People who have been subjected to surgery or who suffer from the effects of injury, or other illness, are not inclined to be ambulant. However, as far as possible, they should be encouraged to get out of bed for some part of the day and, if not, to move their legs in bed. Physiotherapy is an essential adjunct to convalescence and an uncomplicated recovery. A pulmonary embolus following surgery or injury is usually an isolated incident and, once the patient has recovered and is up and about again, is unlikely to recur. However, emboli as complications of other chronic illnesses, such as rheumatic heart disease, are recurring phenomena and should be considered as complications of the chronic disease. Any young woman contemplating taking the contraceptive pill is advised against doing so if she has any history of thrombosis following childbirth since the contraceptive pill is thought to encourage thrombosis and emboli, particularly in those already susceptible. Death from pulmonary embolus has been known in young, previously healthy women who have been taking the pill for some time.

QUINSY

This disease is usually preceded by acute tonsillitis, an inflammation of the tonsils. The inflammation and infection spread to the tissues surrounding the tonsil and abscess formation occurs.

Symptoms include severe sore throat and difficulty with swallowing and some cases have ended fatally due to swelling of throat tissue with blockage of respiratory passages. Pneumonia and haemorrhage are two other serious side-effects that may occur.

This condition can usually be avoided by treating tonsillitis with penicillin or other suitable antibiotics. However, if it does develop, it can sometimes be helped by incision and drainage of the abscess.

RENAL DIALYSIS

When the body is functioning normally a large number of chemical reactions are taking place, which provide energy and during which waste products are formed. Many of these waste substances are removed in the urine by the kidney. Blood flows through the kidneys and substances useless and toxic to the body are filtered off. If kidney function fails the waste products accumulate in the body and finally cause so much pollution that survival is impossible. The main waste product is known as urea, and the other substance which causes serious disturbance if it is not kept within certain limits is potassium.

Kidney failure may be acute or chronic. In either event there are certain individuals who can be treated by means of dialysis and the artificial kidney. Dialysis is the name given to the process of filtration of blood through a filter outside the body. The artificial kidney is the actual filter.

Acute renal failure may occur after severe injury or major surgery when the blood-supply to the kidney is reduced to such an extent that kidney function is lost. Acute kidney disease may also be a cause of acute failure. Very often these cases respond to diet, control of fluid intake, and rest. However, recourse to the artificial kidney is indicated when, despite treatment, the concentration of urea and potassium in the blood rises to levels incompatible with normal body function.

Chronic renal failure occurs over a number of years and may be due to disease or congenital abnormality. Suitable people can be maintained on regular dialysis and be relatively fit and healthy for years.

There are several problems associated with dialysis, including practical and ethical ones. From a practical point of view, numbers of artificial kidneys are limited by financial resources and there are more patients than kidneys. There is a shortage of kidney units and only the major centres have these. People in outlying areas often have to travel long distances to obtain treatment. This may interfere with working time and, although they remain fit, they lose their jobs. Some people have kidney units installed in their homes—at hospital and local authority expense. Others, more materially fortunate, install these machines at their own expense. A kidney machine in the home requires the close co-operation of relatives and the space for installation. People on kidney treatment cannot stray far from their machines since dialysis is required twice per week. The ethical problems consist of the difficulties involved in choosing patients for this treatment. Selection must take into account the personality of the individual and if he or she is temperamentally suitable. The relative importance to society of one person compared to another, i.e., bread-winner, housewife, teenage schoolchild, young man, or old man, has also to be taken into consideration. These are very difficult choices to make and often it is impossible to do so.

People on kidney machines are living, in a sense, on borrowed time and they may feel very insecure regarding the safety of the machine and the ability of relatives, despite vigorous training, to deal with their machines. They will, however, be as they were prior to disease and much better than before treatment, providing that the machine is functioning correctly. The present opinion is that artificial dialysis should be a temporary treatment to be followed at a suitable time by kidney transplant.

RHEUMATIC FEVER

Rheumatic fever is an inflammatory disease which occurs mainly in children and which often has permanent disabling effects. It is more common in the lower social classes and is associated with malnutrition, overcrowding, poverty, and dirt. Although the first attack occurs in childhood there may be recurrent episodes throughout life, each one producing further irreversible damage to body tissues.

The disease is thought to be due to a sensitivity reaction by the body. A sore throat usually precedes an attack of rheumatic fever by 2 or 3 weeks, and it is thought that the bacteria causing the sore throat produce poisons which act on the tissues causing an inflammatory reaction. The main tissues affected are the heart and the joints.

Symptoms include loss of weight and joint pains, often called 'growing pains' by ill-informed parents. These are followed by high temperatures, swollen joints, and severe pain. During this period the child should be confined to bed and treated with aspirin to reduce inflammation and temperature. It is also at this stage that the heart muscle may be affected although this organ is not always injured by the disease.

The main danger of recurrence is further heart damage and, to avoid the danger of this, prolonged rest and supervision are very important. Penicillin is usually given for 5 years following an attack to prevent further bacterial infection and the dose is stepped up for operations such as tonsillectomy or tooth extractions. During these procedures if bacteria are present in teeth and tonsils they are able to enter the blood-stream; high penicillin dosage will kill them before they can do any damage.

There is a tendency for parents of a child who has had rheumatic fever to treat him as a semi-invalid for the rest of his life. This is a very unwise thing to do. The child should gradually return to daily activities until he is leading a normal life again, although he should not be allowed to become fatigued. To make a child an invalid is to deprive him of his natural development pattern. The more serious effects of rheumatic fever may show themselves in middle life. Damage to heart valves in youth makes them incompetent and with increasing age the heart becomes less and less able to function. There is increasing breathlessness and inability to do any kind of work or activity and finally the heart will fail. Operations are now available to repair heart valves and these are fairly successful. Damaged heart valves are liable to infection and subacute bacterial endocarditis is a serious complication and increases the damage to the valve.

Girls with rheumatic fever who have valve damage should not be encouraged to have children. This increases the work of the heart, both during pregnancy and afterwards in rearing. A child whose mother is a semi-invalid is deprived and the loss of a mother at an early age may be damaging to emotional development. A couple contemplating rearing a family should consider the problem from the child's angle before they enter into this difficult and demanding task.

A man who has cardiac valvular disease may find himself prohibited from bread-winning in middle life. Any young man who has had rheumatic fever and has signs of heart damage should be advised to train for a sedentary occupation with an eye to future disability.

RHEUMATOID ARTHRITIS

Rheumatoid arthritis is an inflammatory disease affecting the joints and other tissues. It is liable to occur in all age-groups but is more common in women. There is a form of the disease which occurs in children known as Still's disease. The causative agent is unknown although various factors have been cited, including viral and bacterial poisons. The acute phase of the disease is usually followed by permanent disability of varying degree.

General symptoms include loss of weight and fatigue, loss of appetite, and anaemia. These are followed by swelling and pain of body joints, particularly of the hands. Complications include inflammation of arteries leading to interference with blood-supply and development of pressure-sores and ulcers, damage to nerves leading to loss of sensation and movement in various parts of the body, eye damage, and deafness due to inflammation of the joints between the conducting bones of the middle ear (*see* DEAFNESS).

The acute phase is treated by bed-rest, drugs, adequate diet, and splinting of the affected joints. Drugs include aspirin which has a specific effect in reducing inflammation and pain. Gold injections are still used and they reduce inflammation although gold may cause kidney disease. Cortisone is effective in reducing inflammation and pain but also carries the risk of serious side-effects. As soon as the temperature drops and the acute phase subsides it is important to encourage activity to prevent joint immobility. Physiotherapy and occupational therapy are extremely important in helping to restore function and mobility. Unless the disease is very mild there is going to be residual disability and the person affected must be made aware of this as soon as possible so that adjustment and adaptation may be brought about as quickly as possible. This requires the co-operation and patience of the family and they should understand the nature and extent of the disability. The change may be drastic—reducing a breadwinner to dependence on his wife, and a mother to dependence on her husband and children. There are available many kinds of help including aids to daily living such as cutlery with large handles, tap levers, etc. In addition, houses may be adapted, invalid cars are available for mobility, and there are social clubs for disabled people. Retraining for employment may be necessary. The disease is disfiguring and this may cause some emotional difficulties, particularly in women.

SMALL-POX

This is a severe infectious disease caused by a virus. Although it was originally a disease of the East it now occurs in a world-wide distribution owing to rapid travel and constant immigration. The condition carries a mortality rate of 30 per cent in its severest form.

Symptoms include a high temperature, headache and backache, followed by a drop in temperature and the development of a rash. Secondary infection of the rash can occur and cause further complications. In the most severe form of small-pox the rash is haemorrhagic and death occurs in 3–4 days. Identification of the disease is done by taking a scraping of the rash and inoculating this into eggs to grow the virus.

Infection occurs via the discharges from the rash and also through coughing and sneezing. The virus can also linger on articles belonging to an infected individual and can be carried by another person. A person remains infectious until the rash is completely healed.

A vaccine has been developed which is highly protective. The method of protection in this country is to vaccinate at 18 months and then to follow this with further re-vaccination every 3–5 years. Nurses, doctors, and travellers should be meticulous about vaccination and make sure they are always up to date. The complications of vaccination include virus encephalitis and generalized vaccinia (a mild form of small-pox). People with eczema and asthma should avoid vaccination if possible. Education of the public is important in preventing the rise in incidence of this disease. The sad fact is that, unless an epidemic occurs fairly frequently, people soon forget the horrors of the disease and become lazy about protection. It is only by refreshing memories at frequent intervals that a reasonable level of vaccination is maintained in the community.

When a case occurs it should be notified to the Local Health Authority immediately. The patient should be isolated and all contacts should be vaccinated immediately and kept in quarantine for 16 days following exposure since it takes up to 16 days for the disease to develop. It is important to trace the source of the infection and to break the chain.

Small-pox disfigures and leaves a pitted skin where the rash has been. People who have had small-pox therefore have scarred faces. Recovery gives immunity to further attack.

Immigration from the East increases the danger of small-pox in this country. It is thus important to ensure that every immigrant entering this country has been vaccinated for small-pox, but it is not always possible to be absolutely certain of this fact. Travelling to distant countries is hazardous from the disease aspect and the value of being vaccinated against small-pox cannot be stressed too often, both for protection of individual and community.

SMOKING

Smoking tobacco has been a national pastime in this country for over 300 years. Originally introduced to this country from America there are three main types of the indulgence: the cigarette, the cigar, and the pipe. It is, however, cigarettes which are the great danger to health and have been demonstrated to be a prime cause in the development of lung cancer, as well as an associated factor in other serious diseases.

Cigarettes are on sale freely in this country and, despite the large amount of tax added to the basic price, people continue to indulge. In America a large anti-smoking campaign is in action and all cigarette packets carry the legend 'Dangerous to health'. Smoking may be a social habit or an addiction. Once the habit of inhaling the smoke is developed there is the possibility of addiction and the added risk of the smoke continuously coming into contact with the lung.

The main substances in cigarette smoke thought to cause lung cancer are arsenic and 3:4-benzpyrene. However, there may be others which have not yet been found. It is shown by research that the more cigarettes smoked the higher the chance of cancerous changes. More than twenty cigarettes a day over a number of years increases the risk forty times.

The fact that the relationship between cigarettes and lung cancer has been proved without doubt does not stop people smoking. There are several factors involved. People who feel well never worry about ill health and a cigarette smoker who enjoys his habit will not give up smoking because someone says that it causes disease. He feels all right and he has been smoking like a chimney for many years. Furthermore, smoking has been a tradition in this country for some three centuries and tradition must be maintained at all costs. Some people are truly addicted to smoking and find it so difficult to abstain that, however much they are determined to try, they find that they have to return to the packet. People who are socially insecure find a cigarette a great comfort in any awkward situation. Others use it as a sedative when work pressures mount. Cigarettes are thought to be responsible for the birth of small babies and pregnant women have been asked to avoid smoking. Cigarettes are also thought to cause constriction of blood-vessels and to be an exciting factor in the development of coronary heart disease. They aggravate chronic bronchitis and other chronic chest conditions.

The only way to deal with the problem is prevention of cigarette-smoking. It is essential that children be made aware of the danger of smoking and the ill-effects of developing the smoking habit. Parental example is as important as the words and demonstrations of the professional health educator. However, in the last analysis one can only give accurate information and advice. One cannot prevent people from deliberately injuring themselves if they choose to do so.

SODIUM

This element is essential to normal body function and is contained in the body fluids as sodium chloride or salt. Some sodium is also contained in the bones.

Sodium is found in many foods in normal diet but in most cases it is necessary to add salt to the food in order to provide sufficient for normal body requirement. If the body needs salt a craving may occur and further salt be added to the diet. Excess sodium is excreted by the kidneys in the urine. When excess sodium is lost by other routes, such as heavy sweating, no sodium is lost in the urine.

Sodium balance in the body is controlled by the adrenal cortex. When the cortex is damaged (*see* ADDISON'S DISEASE) large quantities of sodium are excreted leading to sodium depletion and all the other diet symptoms and complications, including low blood-pressure and weakness. Sodium loss accounts for many of the symptoms of Addison's disease. Sodium may also be lost in excess quantities due to damaged kidneys.

Provided that there is sufficient water available the kidney can excrete unlimited quantities of sodium. In the desert, survival is limited because sodium cannot be excreted in sufficient amounts and the effects of sodium excess cause death. Sodium also accumulates due to heart failure and kidney disease.

Sodium depletion is usually associated with dehydration as in excess heat or diarrhoea. Muscle cramps, weakness, vomiting, and loss of appetite are all symptoms of loss of too much sodium from the body.

Sodium accumulation is always associated with excess water retention and oedema. This is usually due to heart failure and kidney disease.

SPINA BIFIDA

Spina bifida is the name given to a congenital condition affecting the spinal column and cord. It is a developmental defect due to unknown causes which gives rise to a swelling in one of several places along the midline of the back. The defect may consist of lack of bone leading to a bulging of the membranes lining the canal, but, in severe cases, the cord is also abnormal and nervous tissue is incorporated into the general swelling. If the swollen bulging area consists of membranes alone it is called a meningocele and is usually covered with skin. If nerves are also included skin is usually lacking and this is called a meningomyelocele. Lack of skin plus the exposure of nervous tissue leads to rapid infection if treatment is not instituted. The defect is most commonly observed in the lower third of the back or lumber region, but it may also be found in the neck region or the chest region. Repair of a simple meningocele is relatively easy and will usually leave no residual damage. However, where nervous tissue is involved, although repair and attempted closure of the defect may remove the swelling, there are always residual, permanent complications. In any case repair should be carried out soon after birth to prevent infection.

Involvement of nervous tissue occurs early in the prenatal development and consequently there is abnormality of function of those parts supplied by the nerves affected. In spina bifida, involvement of nerves leads to paralysis or weakness of the lower limbs. Bladder and bowel paralysis cause double incontinence. The complications of these abnormalities include kidney disease due to back-pressure and infection from a paralysed bladder, pressure-sores, and deformities and fractures of the useless lower limbs. Operations have been devised to relieve back-pressure of urine, mainly by diverting the flow from the bladder to the external abdominal wall. Deformities of the limbs have to be corrected by orthopaedic surgery. Sometimes spina bifida is also accompanied by hydrocephalus (*see* HYDROCEPHALUS).

The problems associated with the survival of a child with severe spina bifida are manifold. Apart from long periods in hospital and numerous surgical and medical procedures, which are painful and unpleasant, there are all the other factors of emotional conflict in the parents with consequent family problems, neglect of other children in the family, the ethics of saving a child with a permanent disability, and the needs and wants of a physically disabled child who is often mentally normal. These factors have already been discussed in relation to cerebral palsy. However, in the case of spina bifida the defect is obvious at birth whereas it is often weeks before cerebral palsy is diagnosed. This may give rise to considerable problems, but unfortunately most parents are ignorant of the implications of this condition and, before they know enough to decide on the fate of the child, the choice is out of their hands. The real question is 'Does the sanctity of human life include the survival of children who are going to spend their lives in pain and discomfort, who are going to be segregated, and whose needs and desires are rarely going to be fulfilled however hard they strive?' By the time a social worker is involved this is irrelevant, but the parents will need a great deal of help and accurate information and they will be interested in the future rather than the past. Any parents of spina bifida children contemplating further family should realize that the risk of having another is increased. Obviously, it is the choice of the parents as to further reproduction but they should be given accurate information.

SYPHILIS

Syphilis is a venereal disease. It is passed from one person to another by sexual contact. Occasionally it is contracted in other ways. A dentist working with a patient who has syphilis may be bitten and develop signs of the disease on his hand. A doctor or nurse may also contract the condition in similar manner. Children may be born with the disease which can be passed on through the placenta from mother to foetus. It is caused by a corkscrew-shaped bacterium called a spirochaete.

The disease occurs in three stages. The primary stage is the chancre, which is a painless sore developing on the sexual organs. It can easily be overlooked in a women although in a man it is usually obvious. As the chancre is developing—it appears 3 weeks after infection—the bacteria are also entering the blood-stream and 6 weeks after infection the secondary stage appears, with all its attendant symptoms. This stage may mimic many diseases and includes rashes of various sorts, headache, temperature, and swollen glands. These symptoms all disappear after a short time.

The tertiary stage may take up to 20 years before it reveals itself. The bacteria enter various organs from the blood-stream and slowly destroy tissue by forming encapsulated areas called gummata. These gummata only appear in the brain, bones, skin, and cardiovascular system. The aorta, which is the large blood-vessel carrying oxygenated blood to tissues from the heart, is particularly affected and areas of the wall of this blood-vessel become very thin and balloon out to form an aneurysm. This may burst at any time and cause sudden death. Gummata in the brain cause dementia of a special kind known as general paralysis of the insane or G.P.I., and symptoms include delusions of grandeur and persecution. Other symptoms include severe abdominal pain, loss of sensation in the feet and legs, and blindness. The tertiary lesions are full of the bacteria.

Special tests for the presence of syphilis include the Wassermann and Lange tests. These utilize the principle of antibody formation by the blood-stream. If the spirochaete is present it provokes the usual antibody response with the production of substances in the blood that are antagonistic towards the organism and tend to destroy it. Identification of these antibodies may indicate syphilis, but it is possible to obtain false-positive results and confirmation should be obtained by finding the bacteria in the blood or the cerebrospinal fluid, or the actual gummata.

Syphilis can be cured by penicillin but this must be given in adequate doses for some time. General control methods should include health education, premarital and prenatal medical examinations. Suppression of prostitution does help to a certain extent. It is important to trace all contacts of an infected case since these will be infected and may pass on the disease to others. It is also important to provide early, accessible treatment which is free.

Syphilis is associated with sexual promiscuity. The incidence always rises during periods of war when soldiers, freed of normal restrictions, make use of available prostitutes and other women to relieve their sexual tensions and loneliness. Poor socio-economic conditions encourage the spread of the disease, but it is also rising in those affluent countries where standards of behaviour are changing and the younger generations are uncertain of their own standards. Sexual freedom always leads to a certain amount of promiscuity and experimentation and, since the last war, the incidence of syphilis has risen in this country, particularly in the younger age-groups. Although treatment has an excellent result, there is still stigma attached to the disease and many people fail to seek medical help. Skilled social work is as important as medical aid in this field.

THRUSH

This infectious disease is caused by a fungus. It is also known as moniliasis. It attacks the lining of various organs of the body and also affects the skin.

The fungus forms white membranous patches on the affected surfaces and a diagnosis may be made by taking a scraping of the membrane and looking at it under a microscope.

It is found everywhere in the world and is particularly common in newborn babies and pregnant women. Common sites for infection are the mouth and vagina. It also causes disease in the lungs, the linings of the brain (meninges), and the heart. It attacks moist skin and infection occurs in obese people in those areas which rub and sweat, e.g., breast folds and thighs. Housewives who are continually putting their hands in water may have finger infections.

If the vagina is infected during childbirth the new infant will be contaminated and develop thrush within 2–5 days. It can also be termed a venereal disease when it is present in the vagina as it can be transmitted via sexual intercourse.

Patients receiving antibiotic treatment may develop monilia. The antibiotics upset the normal bacterial content of the intestine and this allows the fungus to enter the body.

Treatment is simple and effective. Babies with thrush should be isolated until it is cleared. All articles and secretions should be disinfected. The antifungal agent nystatin is used to destroy the fungus. It is given by mouth in liquid or tablet form. Gentian violet, which was in use prior to the development of nystatin, is still used by some doctors and it is still possible to see newborn babies with purple tongues who are being treated for thrush.

Social implications of this disease are minimal and it carries no stigma. If transmitted venereally it is usually from wife to husband and should not cause marital problems.

THYROTOXICOSIS

This is a disease caused by overactivity of the thyroid gland. The gland is situated in the neck and manufactures a hormone, thyroxine, which is responsible for the control of body activity. Thyroxine is formed from iodine which is normally ingested in the diet and removed from the blood by the thyroid.

There is no known cause for the development of overactivity of the thyroid although it is said that emotional stress can be a trigger force. It is more common in women than in men. The gland is enlarged and may contain cysts. Often the most obvious signs are protruding eyes (or exophthalmos).

There are many symptoms including nervousness and irritability, loss of weight, fast pulse, breathlessness, vomiting, and loss of hair. The person may present a startled appearance owing to the effect on the eyes. Bloodpressure may be raised. The basic effect is to increase all tissue activity above normal and the person is in a constant state of overactivity. The most serious complication is that of heart failure. Prolonged overactivity of heart muscle leads to degeneration, heart enlargement, and irreversible damage. Diabetes is another complication which occurs due to prolonged overaction of the pancreas with consequent exhaustion (*see* DIABETES).

Treatment may be medical or surgical. There are drugs which antagonize thyroid activity and can be successful in treating the symptoms of the disease. Radioactive iodine has also been used. All iodine is taken up by the thyroid, including the radioactive variety. In sufficient doses this can destroy thyroid tissue to the point where there is only sufficient left to produce normal activity. Surgical removal of some thyroid tissue has the same effect. However, in some cases too much thyroid tissue is destroyed, by either radioactivity or surgery, and the patient becomes hypothyroid, i.e., is not sufficiently supplied with thyroid hormone. In these cases replacement therapy must be instituted and the individual takes thyroid hormone in controlled doses permanently.

The symptoms of thyrotoxicosis can simulate those of neuroses, and a person showing symptoms of irritability and nervousness and loss of weight must never be regarded as one with psychiatric problems until organic disease is excluded. People who are thyrotoxic may be very difficult and may suffer from psychiatric disturbance before treatment. They are liable to lose their tempers very easily. There is often a heightened libido in women who make extra demands on their husbands and this may cause some marital conflict. Treatment usually relieves all these symptoms, but there is a delicate balance between too much, just enough, and too little thyroxine, and anyone dealing professionally with a person suffering from an overactive thyroid should be aware of possible symptoms and take early steps if these appear.

TUBERCULOSIS

This is an infectious disease caused by an organism known as the tubercle bacillus. There are various forms of this bacterium which affect different species of animals. Only the human and bovine types can infect human beings. Infection by the bacteria causes inflammatory reaction by the body tissues leading to areas of tissue destruction and cavity formation which is a cardinal sign of the disease. Sometimes the tubercle bacilli erode into a blood-vessel and they can then travel rapidly to many parts of the body from the original site of infection. This is known as disseminated or miliary tuberculosis.

Bovine bacillus (affecting cows) is excreted in milk and is an uncommon cause of tuberculosis in this country. However, if it is present it causes abdominal symptoms or miliary tuberculosis. It has almost been eradicated due to slaughter of infectious cattle and pasteurization of milk. Most cases of tuberculosis in this country are caused by inhalation of bacilli spread in the air by the coughing of a person infected with the disease. In the majority of cases the primary site of infection is in the lungs. Many people are infected by tuberculosis in childhood or adolescence. The infection in most cases remains circumscribed and dies down after a short while with no ill effects. The only remaining sign that infection has occurred is a small area in the lung which shows up on X-ray and is a healed tuberculosis lesion containing calcium. This primary infection evokes the antigen–antibody reaction and the presence of specific antibodies in the blood-stream will prevent any further invasion by the tubercle bacillus. In some cases the primary infection leads to serious disease.

Resistance to infection depends on many factors. There is a genetic basis for resistance as has been shown by studies of homes and families. Environmental conditions also play a big part in preventing or encouraging tuberculosis. Overcrowding, poverty, poor working conditions, malnutrition, lack of exercise, and long hours of overwork all help to reduce resistance to the disease. Nutrition is important and regular well-balanced meals play a big part in developing protection against infection. Active immunization (B.C.G.) has also played a large part in reducing the infection rate. The presence of other disease increases the chances of tuberculosis infection and these include schizophrenia, diabetes, and silicosis.

Ninety per cent of tuberculosis cases in this country are of the lung, and the majority of these occur in the elderly rather than the young. Old men living on their own, neglecting themselves, and failing to eat properly are prone to tuberculosis infection. In some cases this is undiagnosed for some time and elderly persons who come into contact with children, such as grandchildren or other young relatives, are likely to infect them and cause severe illness.

Infection of the lungs may be present for some time before symptoms appear. Early symptoms include night sweats, loss of weight and appetite, temperature, cessation of periods, cough with sputum, and coughing of blood. Severe tiredness is a common symptom. Later complications include the spread of bacteria to other tissues both adjacent and widespread, severe haemorrhage, secondary infection with pneumonia, and heart failure.

Treatment is prolonged and consists of bed-rest, good nutrition, good nursing, and the use of modern drugs.

Occasionally it is necessary to resort to surgery with removal of infected and diseased parts of the lung. Exposure to sunlight exacerbates the symptoms and should be avoided. People with tuberculosis must be isolated from those who are uninfected and unprotected.

Active immunization with B.C.G. vaccine (*see* B.C.G.) is a necessity for all staff working with tuberculosis patients. All cases must be followed up for some years after cure since infection often recurs in those who have tissues already damaged by the disease. Return to poor environmental conditions predisposes to further infection. Overwork must be avoided and pregnancy is contra-indicated for 5 years after infection is cured.

People who are not coughing tuberculosis bacilli in their sputum are not infectious to other people. However, there is still a stigma attached to tuberculosis and there are often difficulties with re-employment and social life. Many patients undergoing prolonged treatment in hospitals and sanatoria become very much aware of the disease and identify themselves with it as part of their lives. The closed environment of a hospital becomes secure and sheltering, and going out into the world after 2 or 3 years is an ordeal for many cured individuals. Tuberculosis is being eradicated in the developed areas of the world, but with air travel and immigration the possibility of entry of active cases must not be overlooked and all those exposed to infection should be protected. All schoolchildren are offered active immunization at the age of 14 years, if they have not developed a natural resistance. There is a high acceptance rate since, unlike other infectious disease, tuberculosis is still considered a serious hazard.

ULCERATIVE COLITIS

This is a disease affecting the colon which can occur at any age. The cause is unknown. It used to be considered that emotional upset and conflict were often responsible for deterioration in the disease and possible reasons for its onset. However, the general feeling at present is that emotional upset may be secondary to the disease.

The lining of the colon and rectum is affected. It becomes inflamed with superficial ulcers. The first symptoms are constipation and blood. Diarrhoea is a later problem with faecal incontinence and abdominal cramps.

It is thought that people of a certain personality are prone to colitis. These tend to be timid and overdependent, who lack aggression and are uncertain. However, this may be the result rather than the cause.

There are certain complications of the disease which may be dangerous to life. There may be massive bleeding, perforation into the abdominal cavity, or cancerous changes. Arthritis may also be associated, which may be due to poison produced during the disease process which pours into the blood and affects the joints. Anaemia may be severe from the bleeding.

Occasionally the disease is acute with severe diarrhoea, weight-loss, and high temperature.

Colitis in children stunts growth due to lack of reabsorption of essential substances through the damaged intestine wall.

Pregnancy has an unpredictable effect. It may worsen the disease or cause improvement.

Treatment is by rest, fluid, iron, and drugs. Cortisone is used but great care should be exercised with this drug. Surgery should only be resorted to when the disease becomes disabling, perforation occurs, or to prevent cancer. The surgical procedure consists of excising the diseased bowel and bringing the open bowel-end to the external abdominal wall—known as a colostomy. In some cases the colon may be removed and the small intestine reconnected to the rectum. In most cases the rectum is also affected and this operation is useless.

The problems associated with colostomy should be discussed briefly here. Colostomy means permanent removal of faeces through a hole in the abdominal wall with a plastic bag attachment. People with colostomy worry about smell, overflow, and the general distastefulness of this type of faecal removal. Diet is important since it is important to avoid loose stools. Women are particularly worried about having the operation from the point of view of clothing and marital relationship. It is a difficult decision, but it usually means the difference between severe disability and death and a relatively normal life. It is a decision only the affected person can make and the only thing that the professional person can do is provide the facts.

URTICARIA

Urticaria is a skin response to a variety of agents both external and internal. This response only occurs in certain sensitive individuals and each person responds differently to different agents. The response is due to the release of a substance known as histamine, which causes dilatation of the blood-capillaries and consequent skin redness. Fluid leaks from the capillaries and this causes a local raised white area, or wheal. Severe itching may also occur. Wasp stings and nettles contain histamine and can cause this skin reaction in people who come into contact with either.

Histamine is contained in the skin and other tissues and is released when the agent to which the individual is sensitive is encountered. Previous encounter with this agent has caused the development of antagonistic substances in the blood, and the presence of the antagonist causes release of histamine when it comes into contact with the causative agent. Penicillin and certain foods can cause this reaction as well as plants, certain metals such as nickel, and many other common objects. Individuals prone to asthma and hay fever are particularly likely to develop urticaria.

In many cases of urticaria there is no obvious exciting cause. Emotional stress is said to trigger off urticarial skin response. Giant urticaria is a variety which is inherited. It can be serious since wheals may form in the upper respiratory tract and inhibit respiration.

Urticaria may be treated by local application of antihistamine ointments, by oral administration of antihistamine tablets, and sometimes by reapplying the causative agent and actually desensitizing the individual by a series of injections. If antihistamine drugs are being taken, driving is contra-indicated since a side-effect of these drugs is drowsiness. It is particularly dangerous to take any alcohol when on antihistamine treatment.

VARICOSE VEINS

Varicose veins refer to the dilated and distorted blood-vessels which occur due to prolonged high venous pressure and which are most commonly seen in the legs. Other areas where they may occur are in the rectum (piles or haemorrhoids) or the testicle (varicocele). Varicose veins of the lower limbs can occur in either sex at any age but are particularly common in women, who are more likely to be subject to prolonged high pressure in the veins in association with pregnancy and menstruation.

In man the erect position in itself causes a high venous pressure due to the effect of the pull of gravity. Return of blood from the legs to the heart is effected by active muscular squeezing on the veins during activity. Blood is prevented from running backwards during muscular relaxation by valves in the veins.

The basic problem causing varicosity is defective valves. This may be due to congenital deformity but there is also a heredity factor involved. In other cases abnormal dilatation occurs due to pressure during pregnancy and this distorts and damages veins. Varicose veins may also arise following clotting in the veins with consequent valvular damage. This may occur after childbirth or operations, when pelvic damage and enforced rest encourage blood-clotting.

Symptoms of varicose veins include prominent and disfiguring veins, pain in legs, particularly after standing for some time, itching, irritation, and changes in skin colour.

Complications of varicose veins are due to the fact that blood lies almost static. Fluid leaks out from these vessels and gives rise to swelling (oedema). Lack of blood movement also leads to the development of ulcers, dermatitis, and infection in the affected limbs.

Treatment of this condition depends on the severity and the general state of health of the person afflicted. They are often symptomless, the only reason for consultation being cosmetic. In other cases pain and swelling can be relieved by rest and wearing elastic stockings or bandages. The extra support on the legs helps to improve blood-flow in the veins. In some cases the veins are removed by being obliterated. The channels are blocked by injecting them with a substance which destroys them. The difficulty here is that sometimes the veins become potent again. There are surgical procedures to remove varicose veins and these may be successful, but, often when a varicose vein is removed, varicosity develops in other veins.

Ulcers are treated by rest and support with application of external lotions and ointments. These may include antibiotics if there is any sign of infection. General diet and health measures help to encourage healing.

Varicose veins are a nuisance and can be the cause of much discomfort and limitation of mobility. Obesity can complicate varicosity and those who are overweight should be encouraged to diet. Ulceration is common in elderly people with varicose veins. Blood-flow is important in preventing development of ulcers and mobility should be encouraged in all those with varicosities.

VITAMINS

'Vitamin' is the name given to a group of chemical substances which occurs naturally in foods and which is essential to the maintenance of normal body function. They are required in minute amounts only and there has to be a severe deficiency before ill effects become apparent.

Vitamin-deficiency diseases occur when the diet is unbalanced and usually more than one vitamin is involved, giving rise to a number of signs and symptoms. Vitamins are named alphabetically and each has a specific role in the maintenance of health.

Vitamin A is responsible for the integrity of normal sight and skin texture. Lack of vitamin A leads to night blindness and a dry scaly skin. It is also important for normal growth. It is present in all animal fats and can also be manufactured by the body from a substance called carotene, which is responsible for the colour of carrots.

Vitamin B is a complex of several substances found in vegetable foods, including cereals and pulses. They are also found in liver and meat. Lack of vitamin-B complex may give rise to disturbance of nerve tissue, gastro-enteritis, dermatitis, sore tongue and mouth, and dementia. Lack of cyanocobalamin or vitamin B_{12} is directly responsible for the development of pernicious anaemia.

Vitamin C is a vitamin found in citrus fruits, bread, and potatoes. It is essential to maintain the integrity of the blood-vessel walls and lack of it causes scurvy. It also encourages wound-healing.

Vitamin D is found in fish and is essential for normal bone development. It can also be formed in the skin by the action of sunlight. Lack causes rickets, a bone disease which used to be very common in this country and the resultant effects of which may be seen in people born 50–60 years ago.

Vitamin E is found in vegetable oils. Its function is not yet understood although it is thought to be associated with sterility.

Vitamin K is responsible for the formation of a substance in the liver which is essential for normal blood-clotting. It is found in vegetables.

Vitamin deficiencies are associated with poor social conditions, overcrowding, malnutrition, poverty, old age, and disease. Young children in large poverty-stricken families often suffer from vitamin deficiencies which produce lasting effects on the body, e.g., vitamin D and rickets. Old people living alone often subsist on tea and bread, partly due to lack of resources and partly due to apathy, inability to go shopping, failure to use available services, and food fads. People on strict, self-imposed diets may suffer from vitamin deficiencies if they leave certain things out of the diet. Lack of fresh fruit and vegetables leads to development of scurvy, which in the eighteenth century used to be a common disease of seamen aboard ships for long periods. Now it occurs mainly in the elderly. Parents who are ignorant of the essential nature of vitamins may allow their children to develop certain food fads which will deprive them of certain vitamins. Education is important and advantage should be taken of every opportunity to teach parents accurate facts about food.

WHOOPING-COUGH

This infectious disease is caused by a bacterium. It affects the upper respiratory tract and causes acute and distressing symptoms. It occurs in children and is found in most areas of the world. The disease is spread by bacteria being coughed into the atmosphere or by contact with articles of clothing from infected persons where the bacteria may still be attached.

Symptoms include a cough which becomes severe and is associated with a whooping sound, which gives it its name. It is more infectious before the cough appears, which makes it difficult to control. One attack of whooping-cough produces a strong reaction in the body which will prevent further attacks.

This disease may be prevented to a large extent by active immunization with a vaccine. The vaccine, when injected into the body, stimulates the body to produce substances known as antibodies. These antibodies are chemical substances and are specifically antagonistic to the agent producing them, in this case the whooping-cough bacteria contained in the vaccine. Thus any further exposure to whooping-cough bacteria will provoke an antibody reaction and these antibodies will destroy the bacteria which invade the body. This is part of the normal protective mechanism of the body. Three injections of the vaccine are required to give full immunity. These are usually given in infancy in association with diphtheria and tetanus vaccine and a booster dose is usually advised at 5 years, i.e., school age.

Whooping-cough should be notified to the Medical Officer of Health. Any child who has been in contact with a child with whooping-cough who has not been immunized should be excluded from school and isolated for 7 days.

It is particularly important to protect children who already have chest damage as an attack of whooping-cough may precipitate severe damage and pneumonia. This is done by injecting ready-made antibodies which are immediately effective. However, this is a short-term protection only and vaccination should also be carried out at a later period.

Children with whooping-cough become very tired and irritable from coughing and may also tire a parent considerably. As the condition may last 1–5 months this is a prolonged period of anxiety and weariness and a mother in particular needs a lot of help, both practically and morally.

It is important to educate the public about the importance of protection against whooping-cough and other infectious diseases. A high rate of immunization in the community leads to eradication of the disease in epidemic form. In this country no one is forced to submit his child to any vaccination procedure and many parents who are ignorant about infectious disease and their possible consequences fail to give the protection that is freely available. It is up to the professional staff to give accurate information to parents so that they have a choice of action.

YAWS

This is an infectious disease which occurs in many tropical areas and which causes chronic ill health. The bacterium causing the damage is corkscrew-shaped and physically indistinguishable from the bacterium causing syphilis. It can only be distinguished by immunological investigation. The Wassermann and Kahn tests, so valuable in the diagnosis of syphilis, are also positive in yaws and, because of this, the possibility of yaws must be excluded before syphilis is diagnosed. Yaws is not a venereal disease. It is passed on by direct physical contact with the ulcers of an infected person.

The symptoms arise in three stages. Initially a small raised area appears at the site of the infection which enlarges and looks like a raspberry. After a period of time there are widespread numbers of these raised papules. Finally, they all break down and produce ulcers, particularly on the face and palate. Other complications include bone deformities and secondary infections. The disease is easily and completely cured by a 5-day course of penicillin.

This tropical condition has become important since the beginning of immigration from tropical areas to this country and also widespread international travel, particularly by air. Positive syphilis tests should always take yaws into consideration and a careful history should be taken to elicit past tropical trips or contact with infected persons. Persons who originate from tropical areas should always be considered to have yaws with the symptoms described until proved otherwise. As this is not a venereal disease the dangers of spread are reduced. However, it is more likely to occur in conditions of overcrowding, poverty, and malnutrition, and it is these basic defects in society that should be remedied.

YELLOW FEVER

This is an acute infectious disease caused by a virus. The virus is spread by a mosquito which exists in certain areas of the world. In these areas the disease is said to be endemic, i.e., always present. The mosquito bites man and in the bite is mosquito saliva and virus. The virus enters the blood-stream where it remains for 3 days. It then enters the liver and the main symptoms are due to the results of liver damage.

Symptoms include fever, jaundice, vomiting, headache, and multiple haemorrhages from different parts of the body. Death occurs in 25 per cent of those affected.

There is no specific treatment. Nursing and the administration of fluids are essential. If renal failure occurs the patient must receive artificial kidney treatment.

Due to increase in international air traffic strict watch is necessary to prevent spread of the disease. All those travelling to areas endemic for yellow fever have to be vaccinated every 4 years. The aeroplanes are sprayed to kill any mosquitoes. In many areas yellow fever has been wiped out owing to wholesale attack on the mosquito with D.D.T. and vaccination of whole communities. It is still important to use a mosquito net when sleeping in areas where the disease still occurs.